FIGHT FAT WITH FAT™

2nd edition,
new information, more recipes

Dr. John P. Salerno, Board Certified Family Practice
Complementary Medicine

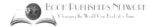
BOOK PUBLISHERS NETWORK
Changing the World One Book at a Time

Book Publishers Network
P.O. Box 2256
Bothell • WA • 98041
Ph • 425-483-3040
www.bookpublishersnetwork.com

BaconFreak.com http://baconfreak.com/ is the ultimate online bacon super-store. They sell three dozen varieties of gourmet bacon, including nitrate-free bacon and thick-cut artisan bacon, as well as bacon jerky. Find more original recipes on their blog, http://BaconToday.com/

This book is intended solely for informational and educational purposes and not as personal medical advice. Please consult your doctor if you have any questions about your health.

10 9 8 7 6 5 4 3 2
Printed in the United States of America

LCCN 2014932470
ISBN 978-1-940598-24-6

Editor: Julie Scandora
Cover Designer: Laura Zugzda
Typographer: Marsha Slomowitz

Contents

PREFACE

John P. Salerno

I owe an enormous debt of gratitude to the late, great Dr. Robert Atkins who was my boss, my mentor, and my friend. I worked in his office as a young doctor and saw with my own eyes the value of the protocols he developed—first to help people with heart disease, and then, almost as if by accident, to help people lose weight.

What did Atkins really say? He said that a low-carb diet could help treat heart disease and help people lose weight. He was right.

But since I started out in his office, our environment has changed dramatically, and the changes significantly affect the food we eat—and our health. In the last twenty years, the food supply in the United State has degraded, and with it, obesity and other lifestyle ailments, including diabetes, heart disease, cancer, and Alzheimer's, have gotten much, much worse.

It is as if our very environment—the food, the water, the air, all that we take for granted—has become poisoned.

In order to save our own lives and the planet, we must adopt sustainable practices at the table. This means understanding that our health depends on sustainable agriculture products and practices and public policy that support health.

In 2010, I went to Washington, DC, to testify before the USDA about the proposed food pyramid. I said what I believe, that the FDA has corrupted the process of formulating the food pyramid and has made recommendations to Americans that do not support health.

Now, I am encouraged to note that a significant body of scientists has signed on to form a committee agreeing with my position—that Americans must be provided with a safer, more nourishing food supply. Our very lives depend on it.

So many issues can interfere with our health and well-being. This fact was brought home to me, up close and personal, when I volunteered at ground zero after 9-11. I began treating people who had volunteered to help in the dreadful task of picking through the rubble, hunting for survivors after the attack on the World Trade Center. Some of those hapless souls have become my patients, and I have cared for them ever since.

So what can the ordinary person do to protect himself? Eat organic produce. Choose wild-caught fish and grass-fed beef. Drink filtered water (and not from a plastic bottle). Purify the air in your home if you live in a polluted area.

These precautions will help to normalize your weight, improve your health, and make for a long and glorious middle age. If Dr. Atkins were alive today, he would agree since he knew the connection between what we eat and the health of our bodies.

To achieve that goal of a healthy life, we must exercise our true power in the marketplace. We begin by being aware of what we put into our mouths. Then we act upon that awareness by choosing wisely. We reject GMO foods, industrial farming, and confined-animal feeding operations and provide a healthier dinner table for ourselves and our children.

The power to create the environment we need for a healthy life rests with each one of us.

ACKNOWLEDGMENTS

I would like to thank the many people in my life who have been so important to me in creating this book.

First, I would like to thank my brother Louis for his always brilliant advice and caring. He has given me the inspiration and shown me the work ethic I needed to be successful.

I would also like to thank my wonderful parents, John and Louise, who have always nurtured me with love and support beyond words.

My wife, Helene, and my nine-year-old son, John, and five-year-old daughter, Sophia, have always been there for me and have lent their unconditional support and love. My children now remind me what is bad for me to eat. John is an avid cyclist, who rides with me every morning, rain or shine. It is on these special rides where I have received perhaps the best insight for my book from a child's perspective. Sophia, the aspiring artist and dancer, has given me ideas for the importance of developing healthy taste buds at an early age and is also quick to remind me to give her daily vitamins.

Lastly, Aunt Josie was my inspiration to take vitamins at an early age and is always there for me.

TOP TEN QUESTIONS ABOUT FIGHT FAT WITH FAT DIET

1. How is the Fight Fat with Fat Diet different from Atkins?

When Dr. Atkins developed his protocols some thirty years ago, we consumed more nutritious food than we do now. Unfortunately, due to the increase in processed foods, proliferation of junk foods, and our degraded farmland, the Atkins protocols just will no longer work.

We have to take a more proactive stand to preserve our health and weight. I find my patients' bodies need a rest from the assaults of the Western diet, and I believe this is true for all of us. A short period, say two weeks, of complete relief from carbohydrates of all types will make it possible to change your life, reset your body clock, and put you on the road to health and long life.

2. Can I eat in a restaurant?

This is the good news. Even in the detox phase of the diet, you can eat out. Skip the French fries, take the burger out of the bread, and enjoy it. Eat grilled fish, roasted chicken, pot roast, tenderloin of pork, shrimp, scallops, pâtés. Any of these work fine in a restaurant at any phase of the diet.

3. What can I eat on the road, at the office, or on the run?

Plan ahead. Boil eggs and keep them on hand for car trips, office snacks, lunches on the run. Lay in a supply of jerky, salmon, nuts of any kind, string cheese. Any of these nutrient-dense foods will keep you satisfied and on track.

4. Vegetables are not in the detox phase. Is this really healthy?

The notion that we have to eat vegetables every day is new. Even as recently as a hundred years ago, mankind had vegetables only during the growing season. To go for a short period with no vegetables is natural and healthy and actually rests your body.

People have been on this earth for thousands of years. We have eaten the same foods twelve months a year for only about a hundred years. Do not worry. Give your body a rest. The detox will take five to fifteen pounds off, reduce your waist size, and more important, rest your overstressed liver and pancreas.

5. Where can I find appropriate food?

We recommend buying food as "close to the ground" as possible, that is whole foods, which have not been treated with chemicals, processed, or mixed with unnatural additives. In the grocery store, choose organic produce, eggs, and dairy. At the farmer's market, ask the vendors how they grow their crops. Find a local provider for meats and fish if possible.

6. Will I ever be able to eat a piece of cake?

As your health becomes more vigorous, you lose weight, and you increase your activities, beginning with a walking regimen of ten thousand steps a day, you will be able to eat more carbohydrates. And, yes, you can even have an occasional piece of cake.

7. How do I balance preparing my special foods with what I need to fix for my partner and children?

Please do not prepare a special meal for yourself. Everyone in the family should be eating a broad and varied diet of unprocessed foods. Your partner and children may kick about it, but if you retain a positive attitude, they will come on board, and every one of you will be healthier.

8. How much weight can I expect to lose?

I have patients who are thrilled to lose twenty pounds. I have patients who have lost upwards of two hundred pounds with no pills and no pain, just learning to love a broad and varied diet of unprocessed foods.

9. When do I go off the diet?

You are never going off the diet. You are making decisions to take care of your body by eating great food for the rest of your life. And if you ever feel your weight creeping back up, give yourself a week of Dr. Salerno's Detox, and you will reset your clock and be back on target in no time.

10.   Tell me one more time. Why should I eat fat?

Natural fat is the most nutrient-dense food there is. It lubricates your joints and is the element that makes your brain work best. It keeps your hair shiny and your skin unwrinkled.

Once you remove the unhealthy processed carbohydrates from your diet, you do not need to worry about natural fat. And perhaps the best part of eating plenty of natural fat is that it is nature's appetite suppressant. Pay attention to your body, and your body will take care of you.

INTRODUCTION

We have virtually eradicated polio, measles, and other devastating diseases, made childbirth significantly safer for both mothers and infants, and saved countless lives with antibiotics. Likewise, dramatically lower rates of infectious diseases, including tuberculosis, rheumatic fever, influenza, and periodontal disease mean that today's children, unlike their peers seventy years ago, can expect to survive beyond their first few years.

However, the United States is on the verge of a health crisis of monumental proportions. These and other impressive medical victories are now being undermined by a bevy of health problems, many of our own making. For the first time, children born today are likely to have a shorter lifespan than their parents, thanks to damage that will be wrought by the terrible trio of obesity, diabetes, and Alzheimer's.

Our genes undeniably play a role in our health and longevity; nonetheless, up to 80 percent of disease is the result of environmental forces.

I use the term "environmental" in the broadest sense to include lifestyle choices we can control. These include what we eat, whether we consume alcohol or smoke, how physically active we are, even the household products we use, as well as those largely beyond our control—including but not limited to industrial toxins in the air and water and pesticides that contaminate and weaken the soil.

We are beginning to pay the price for our disregard for the environment, not just in terms of global warming—devastating as that is—but also in our own health and that of our children. The facts are:

- The actual lifespan of Americans who survive infancy has not changed in more than sixty years.
- Sixty-five percent of American adults are overweight or obese.
- Diabetes has become epidemic in the United States and is on the rise throughout the world.

Even as our bodies are burdened with an increasingly greater toxic burden, we are less able to defend ourselves against assault, weakened as we are by the standard American diet. And now, we are exporting this unhealthful way of eating to the rest of the world.

The multiple reasons for the decline in our overall health are reflected in these facts:

- There are more than one hundred thousand chemicals in regular use in the United States, with an additional seven new ones approved every day.
- Infants are born with almost three hundred chemicals in their blood.
- Our bodies contain hundreds of toxins, including some—such as DDT—that were banned thirty years ago.
- Common pesticides and other chemicals that mimic hormones are implicated in the sharp rise of genital abnormalities in infants and low sperm counts in men.
- According to the US Geological Survey in a 2002 study of stream water samples, 69 percent contained detergents and 66 percent contained disinfectants. The oceans—and

their fish—are contaminated with heavy metals and other toxins.

- Our factory-farm-raised meat and dairy products are laced with growth hormones and antibiotics. Much of the soil in which crops are grown is depleted of vital nutrients, such as calcium, phosphorus, iron, selenium, chromium, and riboflavin.

Therein lies a double whammy: Not only are our air, water, and soil increasingly toxic, but also our food supply, which would normally protect our bodies from toxins, lacks the nutrients to do the job. To compound the problem, our diet is increasingly dominated by foods without much nutritive value, other than calories—fast foods, especially foods full of white flour, sugar, and other refined carbohydrates, as well as trans fats, which may actually do more harm than good as a diet staple.

Most industrialized countries have eliminated hunger as a public health problem, only to have it replaced with another dangerous condition: obesity.

And ironically, people who subsist on doughnuts, bagels, cheeseburgers, potato chips, pizza, soft drinks, and other junk food may be undernourished, even though they are well upholstered.

Obesity and starvation are two sides of the same coin.

According to one Harvard study, the average American eats only three servings of vegetables and fruit a day, a mere one and a half cups, while nine servings, or four and a half cups, are optimal. Shortchanging the diet in such a serious way means missing out on the natural sources for many vitamins and minerals.

Traditional cultures worldwide and over time have gathered whole, unprocessed foods, grown close to home and cooked in simple ways, to produce meals that taste good and nourish the body and the soul. A healthy ration of natural animal fats, including generous portions of saturated fats, have been proven in numerous studies since the 1920s to have salutary effects on everything from brain function to cancer.

Over the past thirty years, Americans have been bombarded by a food industry that threw out theses common-sense notions and turned the family farm into a feedlot. This, in turn, led to a depletion in the quality of animal meat, as well as the soil itself. Then the pharmaceutical industry stepped in to help, offering up an ever more complicated array of solutions to all of the ills that followed, including the introduction of food-like substances that neither nourish nor satisfy.

The food industry and pharmaceutical industry have been telling Americans that low-fat diets are best for their health. That is, quite simply, a lie.

You can see the result on any street in America today. We are the fattest of the Western countries. Ironically, most of the diseases that plague us in the twenty-first century—specifically, heart disease, diabetes, obesity, many forms of cancer, and even Alzheimer's—are associated with excess consumption. Excess intake of white flour, sugar, other refined carbohydrates, and trans-fats are the culprits that rob us of our health, stamina, and long life.

Nutrition is the stepchild of the medical establishment, which focuses on treating illness after the fact, usually with expensive drugs—each with its long list of side effects—rather than on prevention through eating well. This continues, despite the fact that statistics published by the American Medical Association show that 73 percent of all diseases are directly related to nutrition.

Meanwhile, the drug industry experiences peak health, stimulated by expanding markets for new products. Government agencies and health organizations, like the American Cancer Society, routinely state that the causes for most of the disease they represent are unknown.

And so the elephant in the living room continues to go unmentioned. This conscious blindness of the role of the diet and the environment is akin to a refusal to acknowledge the reality of global warming.

The evidence cannot be ignored. Men's average sperm count has declined by about one-third over the last thirty years. A male resident of the United States is eight times more likely to die of prostate cancer than a man in Japan.

We have treated our planet like a garbage dump, and now the toxins are coming home to roost—in our bodies and the bodies of our unborn children. It turns out that when a person experiences genetic damage as a result of a toxin the defective gene can be passed on to the succeeding generations.

The prognosis may sound grim, but I firmly believe there is a solution, and a relatively simple one at that. The very technology that has polluted our planet can also provide us with the know-how to undo past mistakes and avoid similar ones in the future.

There is a tremendous body of research on the processes and chemicals that weaken the body and allow disease to take hold, as well as the role that nutrients play in fortifying the body against disease or even turning back the process of disease. We can harness that knowledge to counter both environmental assaults and genetic weaknesses.

Because I have satellite practices in Japan and Brazil in addition to The Salerno Center in New York, I have the opportunity to compare a culture that has been industrialized for three-quarters of a century with ones that, until recently, were primarily rural. All too many of my foreign patients now suffer from the same diseases that have plagued Americans for decades, strongly suggesting environmental influences.

My understanding of the healing power of nutritious food and the health risks inherent in refined and processed foods was honed working side by side with Dr. Atkins. Many of his long-term patients are now my patients, and I can see the impact that his dietary approach has had on their health. Many are getting on in years but are still remarkably vigorous and free of disease, due, no doubt, to decades of following his low-carb, high-nutrient protocol, all clinically validated in their medical records.

Drawing upon my own clinical experiences in nearly twenty years in family practice and those of other complementary physicians, as well as a vast body of medical research, I have developed a strategy to regulate your weight and decrease your chances of developing cancer, heart disease, diabetes, and other devastating diseases. I call it the Fight Fat with Fat Diet. By putting only good food and water into your body and regularly removing toxins, you can, to a large extent, take charge of your health and live a long, vital, and vigorous life.

The scientifically proven program challenges conventional wisdom on diet, weight control, and disease with a proactive approach to nutrition. The Fight Fat with Fat Diet, a lifestyle plan, offers many benefits:

- immediate and safe weight loss
- radically changed blood chemistry
- halt in adult-onset (type 2) diabetes
- reduction in the risk of a heart attack, stroke, and Alzheimer's and Parkinson's diseases
- no need for calorie counting

The diet is based on eating real unprocessed foods with plenty of fat and protein to regulate bodily functions, control hunger, and prevent cravings. By controlling insulin levels, the body can properly burn sugars, rather than store them as fat, particularly in the midsection, the so-called belly fat. Once you begin to understand portions, you can choose from a healthy assortment of meat, fish, eggs, full-fat cheeses, oils, and nuts without the need to count calories. Then, as you allow your body to regulate itself normally, you can begin to enjoy most vegetables, fruits, and even small amounts of complex carbohydrates, like whole grains and certain sweets.

The Fight Fat with Fat Diet lets diners experience food as it was meant to be enjoyed, in the company of friends and family. People who accept the tenets of this revolutionary plan will no longer look at food as medicine, or something to be endured. They will relish their meals because they will be eating real food, well prepared, and served with joy.

Children's lives can be saved by making a conscious choice right now to stop buying junk food, eating in fast food restaurants, and stuffing their innocent mouths with fake food that can doom them to lives with diabetes, high blood pressure, and perhaps, cancer and heart disease.

My patients, some of whom began with Dr. Robert Atkins, are living proof that one can eat plenty of natural fats, protein, wholesome vegetables, fruits, nuts, and grains prepared in time-honored methods and live long and vigorous lives. And the bottom line is it is an easy protocol to follow—there is no pain or punishment involved.

The Fight Fat with Fat Diet can save lives and change the way America eats.

My goal in this book is to show you how making some simple but profound changes in your daily life can dramatically boost your chances for remaining—or becoming—healthy, despite the toxic soup in which we stew. Against such a challenge, three squares and a daily multivitamin will not give you the defensive edge you need.

How the Diet Works

If you have been eating the normal American diet, most likely, two things have happened: Your weight has crept up, and your energy has gone down. I want to make one thing clear. It is not your fault you are fat. For the past thirty years, you have been pelted with more fake facts, fake foods, and fake science than at any time in the history of mankind. But you can turn that around, starting with this book.

If you walked into a doctor's office now complaining that you are overweight, a good doctor would test your blood to see if you had elevated blood sugar, also known as blood glucose. Your blood glucose level is considered normal if it is below 100, prediabetic if between 100 and 125, and diabetic if over 125. If you are at least fifteen pounds overweight, your blood glucose levels are probably over the normal reading.

If your blood glucose levels are over 100, your body has made a serious maladaptation to a diet with too many processed carbohydrates and sugars. Your cells, which rely on the energy released by the glucose that is made from the normal digestion process, may not be able to process that glucose because you have become insulin resistant.

Insulin is a hormone produced by the pancreas that unlocks the glucose for use by the cells in your body. All energy, whether for movement, thinking, or building your body, depends on a balance between the glucose produced by your digestion and the insulin released by your body.

But things get out of whack when you take in too many over-processed carbs. Glucose goes up and down wildly throughout the day. If you eat cold cereal or a bagel for breakfast, you may find yourself famished only an hour or so later. Some people with severe insulin resistance will get clammy and sweaty. Their heart may pound. All of these are symptoms of blood glucose levels that have become unstable, or hypoglycemic.

We gain weight because insulin becomes elevated from a diet loaded with high carbs: foods with high fructose corn syrup, white flour, and sugars, such as soda pop, donuts, and other highly processed convenience fare. All of these enemies tell the body to store fat.

To regain control of your bodily functions, you need to shock your system by removing all carbohydrates for a short period—about two weeks. I call this the Full Fat Fast. This is not as hard as it sounds, and the results will astound you.

By following this simple plan, my patients have lost anywhere from five to fifteen pounds. They discover, on about day three, that their energy level suddenly zooms up. Within two weeks, their skin begins to glow, their hair begins to shine, and even their nails grow faster. They no longer suffer that mid-afternoon slump when all they want is a nap. Their clothes may feel suddenly loose, and their waist has gone down a couple inches.

When you give the Fight Fat with Fat Detox Full Fat Fast a chance, you will have begun the road to excellent health and optimum weight. In this phase, you subscribe each day to five small meals with full fats. You eat nothing but real food, preferably organic meats, fish, poultry, sausages, full-fat cheeses, and eggs. Because the days of eating chemically laden, hormone-laced fake foods are over, you may have to change the way you shop and start visiting the local farmer's markets and whole-food stores.

Bouts of constipation can be stopped by eating about three tablespoons fiber-rich shirataki, such as Miracle Noodle, with meals or as a snack with a carb-free salad dressing.

Once you move to the next phase—what I call the Marathon—you will be eating a broad and varied array of organic and whole meats, fish, poultry, eggs, vegetables, fruits, and grains. This is a traditional diet, not unlike one that was practiced in countries around the world before the advent of industrial farming.

What you will not be eating are so-called health or diet foods, and certainly no overly processed foods. You will be eating real food, and your body will be grateful. At this point, making a conscious effort to up your fat intake will yield remarkable results. Your weight will go down, your blood chemistry will improve, and your waist size will shrink.

But Fat Makes Us Fat, Right?

No, it does not. The reason your weight is elevated is that your body has converted glucose in your body to stored fat. It has been confused by the typical American diet, which is loaded with sugars, processed carbohydrates, and in many cases, junk food.

On the other hand, I have treated people who believed they were doing the healthiest thing possible by becoming vegetarians or vegans, and yet, their bodies did not lie. Some were overweight. Some had elevated blood glucose levels. Some even had full-blown diabetes type 2. And all they had done was eat vegetables and fruits, often only organic.

How could this have happened?

Some vegetables and many fruits are nature's sugars. While fruits and vegetables have high nutrient values, their natural sugars, added to the other carbohydrates in the diet, will overwhelm our already-stressed systems and produce insulin resistance, particularly the wrong kinds, like carrots, pineapples, grapes, and watermelon. Others, such as corn and peas, also have a high content of natural sugars because, like any seed in nature, they must, by design, be packed with sugars so the seed can develop. These foods need to be avoided, at least at first, if you wish to change your life and improve your health.

When you begin the Marathon, at first you will be restricted to green, leafy vegetables and the cruciferous vegetables, for example, arugula, bok choy, broccoli, Brussels sprouts, cabbage, cauliflower, collard greens, mustard greens, radishes, and watercress. During this period, you will avoid vegetables that grow underground—all of the root vegetables, such as onions, parsnips, carrots, potatoes, which are, by their very nature, high in sugar.

We know the human body is amazingly resilient, and if you just give it half a chance, it can and will recover. Over more than twenty years of medical practice,I have seen this happen in my clients, many of whose weight was completely out of control. I have treated patients successfully who had failed on many other diets: low fat, a range of gimmicky one-ingredient diets (grapefruit, avocado, cabbage, et al.), Weight Watchers, Jenny Craig. Most of these low-fat diets are doomed to fail, whereas this plan puts these patients on the right track for a new way of life.

People can change. You can change. And when you do, you will quickly discover you will never be hungry on this diet. You will never feel that faint, clammy, desperate feeling that signals hypoglycemia again because your body will have plenty of energy at the ready, stored from a steady supply of fat in the diet to get you through the day. You will be eating real food.

The Atkins Connection

Thirty years ago, Dr. Robert Atkins introduced to the world the concept of low carbs and their positive effect on weight loss. His diet worked for millions of people who lost weight and gained energy.

However, after inheriting the Atkins Center's patients and continuing Dr. Atkins's work, I see many many patients today who have difficulty losing weight with the traditional Atkins approach.

Why is this?

The food supply in America has changed for the worse since Dr. Atkins did his groundbreaking work. Our society now has more empty foods, more junk foods, more fast foods, and more fake foods than Dr. Atkins ever could have imagined. It is as if we have forgotten what real food looks like or tastes like.

All my patients are required to do a glucose tolerance test with insulin, and I note a very striking and consistent phenomenon. Many more patients have exceedingly high insulin levels that remain stuck; they do not respond to traditional treatment. These levels that refuse to budge are a direct result of eating too many sugars and refined carbohydrates, including many hidden sugars in processed foods (such as high fructose corn syrup, which appears in almost every prepared food in the marketplace today). It is truly insidious and dangerous.

The modern eater must read labels zealously to ensure consumption of only healthy food. For example, a bottle of cranberry juice cocktail that proudly trumpets no high fructose corn syrup overshadows what it does contain. The fine print reveals that after water, cane sugar is the next ingredient. This sort of three-card monte in the food business tends to confuse even the best-intentioned consumers.

As a result of the difference in foods offered in the marketplace today versus thirty years ago, patients cannot lose weight on Atkins Induction, the first phase of the Atkins Diet, as they did previously.

During this same period, people have stopped cooking from scratch and have begun eating out more often and buying more convenience foods. Some statistics say that people eat out more than 50 percent of the time. And when they buy foods in the marketplace, they tend to be the value-added food products, those ready for consumption and laden with chemicals and highly processed ingredients. This means there are so many hidden sugars, carbohydrates, and chemicals in the diets of most Americans that they do not even know what they are putting into their mouths much of the time.

Only when patients go on the Fight Fat with Fat Diet, beginning with the Full Fat Fast, the regimen of high fat and no carbs, do they see a decrease in insulin with the resulting weight loss. This first phase prepares patients for the long-range change in their eating habits, called the Marathon.

Sometimes patients approach the Full Fat Fast with trepidation, thinking that it is unhealthy not to eat vegetables. But we have had vegetables year round only recently in our long history on Earth. Ancient man routinely went through the winter with no vegetables or fruits at all.

**Our bodies have a deep and ancient understanding of a fat
fast—it is how mankind was able to survive. Trust your body.
It often knows better than you do what you need.**

After the initial detoxification in the Full Fat Fast, complex
carbohydrates are reintroduced slowly, beginning with leafy
vegetables, and later, berries, beans, and seeds, and finally whole
grains. This is a diet easy to follow and embraces the wisdom of
our forebears who ate almost no processed foods and were lean
and healthy for most of their lives.

The modern Western diet that has dominated our choices in
the market has created poor eating habits in the population and a
rise in health problems. We know from experience that the Fight
Fat with Fat Diet will interrupt this cycle and change lives.

Why I Recommend Organic Foods

On the Fight Fat with Fat Diet, you eat nutrient-dense foods, so
the soil in which they grow has a large impact on the vitamins
and minerals. You have to begin with the dirt. The overuse of
pesticides, herbicides, and other chemical additives for the growth
of monocultural, genetically modified crops, including corn, soy,
sugar beets, rice, canola, and others, has wreaked havoc with the
soil. These grain and bean crops grown in this sterile soil not
only are used to create overly processed foods but also are the
basis for animal feed for factory-farmed meats and farm-raised
fish. To compound the problem, because the soil and its products
lack the nutrients they would otherwise naturally have, industry
must add them back in. So in go chemicals to replace the natural
goodness that has been lost. The results are food products with
empty calories and unknown long-term health effects.

They also have the almost certain capacity for making people fat.
Why is this?

Our ancient wisdom says we should eat until we are satisfied, and these foods simply do not satisfy us. Plus, the additives in processed food, which make up for the nutrient loss from chemical-dependent farming practices, create a real problem. These food additives with unpronounceable names and unknown derivatives are known categorically as excitotoxins. Did you ever wonder why Dad could sit down in front of the television to watch the ball game and eat an entire package of corn chips? The Dr. Strangelove additions designed in the lab make that food so tasty, so Dad's natural satiety switch is turned off. Those added chemicals even show up on fresh non-organic produce by way of sprays and dips and chemical baths, further derailing any weight-loss program.

Chemicals can increase food cravings, cause water retention, and actually cause weight gain. These same additives are often allergenic and can cause insulin to spike, playing havoc with those people who are prediabetic or diabetic.

When I go back to Italy, where my family is from, I am amazed at how much better the food tastes. Europe does not permit genetically modified crops, or as a rule, support factory farming. Therefore, you can see with your own eyes that fewer people are overweight and experience for yourself that the food just plain tastes better.

PART I

DIABETES, DIET, AND GOOD HEALTH

DEFINING DIABETES

Diabetes mellitus types 1 and 2 are diseases that prevent your body from properly using the energy from the food you eat.

Type 1 diabetes occurs when the pancreas (an organ behind your stomach) produces little insulin or no insulin at all. Type 1 diabetes, also known as juvenile diabetes, can develop at any age, but it most commonly appears in children, adolescents, and young adults and is a result of a malfunctioning pancreas.

Type 2 diabetes results from a pancreas that has been exhausted by a bad diet and lack of exercise. Type 2 can be thought of as a lifestyle disease that occurs because an improper diet and lack of exercise to create a situation wherein the pancreas makes insulin, but the insulin does not work as it should. This condition is called insulin resistance.

At its most simple, diabetes is a disorder of the glucose metabolism. In plain English, this means that you have diabetes when your body is unable to quickly and efficiently deal with blood sugar (glucose) produced from the breakdown of carbohydrates and other foods.

Consider the classic American dinner of macaroni and cheese casserole with a side salad. The noodles, cheese, milk-based sauce, and breadcrumbs are full of carbohydrates, along with fat and protein. The salad vegetables contain more carbohydrates, as does the salad dressing—along with fat.

The starchy carbohydrates in the noodles and bread crumbs begin to break down into glucose almost the minute you put them in your mouth—the salad vegetables take longer to turn to glucose—and the process is completed in your digestive system. (Protein and fat break down more slowly.)

Your body functions within a fairly narrow blood-sugar-level range, so as highly processed carbohydrate foods begin to convert to glucose and your blood-sugar level rises, your pancreas releases the hormone insulin.

The job of insulin is to ferry blood sugar from your blood stream to your cells, where it can be converted to energy. Any extra blood sugar is converted to glycogen and stored in the liver and muscle cells for use later.

When the glycogen storage areas are full, the remaining glucose is stored as body fat. With fuel for immediate energy needs, plus two auxiliary storage areas—glycogen for the short term and body fat for the long term—this backup system allowed early man to survive for reasonably long periods when food was in short supply.

Obviously, things have changed over the millennia. For most of us, the closest we ever get to a period of famine is the twelve or so hours between dinner and breakfast. Nor do we expend vast amounts of energy traveling everywhere by foot, tracking game, and trying to keep warm without central heat.

So, in our modern times, the converted carbs get stored up for situations that never arrive. Too many carbs will tax your pancreas, and that can lead to type 2 diabetes.

Progression of Diabetes

Let's look at the sequence of events that lead to diabetes.

Step 1: Insulin Resistance

The typical diet in the United States and increasingly in other industrialized countries consists of an excessive number of calories, often in the form of processed food—meaning primarily refined carbohydrates, which quickly convert to glucose. As long as you continue to eat this way, your body never needs to burn its fat for energy. The first sign that diabetes may be in your future is your expanding waistline.

Most people see extra pounds as a cosmetic issue, but they can also gradually make you insulin resistant. That means that your cells are less responsive to the effects of insulin. It is important to state that not everyone with insulin resistance is overweight; nor is everyone who is overweight becoming insulin resistant, but the two are often associated. Why insulin resistance happens is not completely understood, but inflammation appears to play a role.

Step 2: Insulin Resistance with Hyperinsulinism

Because insulin is less effective in making the cells take up the glucose and thereby normalize the blood-sugar level, the pancreas releases more of it, resulting in elevated levels of insulin in the bloodstream.

Instead of the normal rise and fall of both blood-sugar and blood-insulin levels that occur after a meal, the balance has been disturbed. An individual now has both insulin resistance and hyperinsulinism, meaning that after each high-carbohydrate meal, glucose levels rise, prompting a large spike in insulin.

Step 3: Insulin Resistance, Hyperinsulinism, and Low Blood Sugar

As time passes, the mechanism linking insulin and blood sugar becomes increasingly inefficient. It takes longer for the pancreas to produce insulin after a meal and then it overproduces, causing the blood sugar level to drop precipitously when a heavy dose of insulin finally kicks in.

The result, called reactive hypoglycemia, or low blood sugar, can kick off a number of symptoms, such as peaks and valleys in energy, jitters, irritability, and even brain fog. Cravings for sweets and other carbohydrate foods are also common as the body tries to elevate its blood sugar.

Step 4: Prediabetes

Step 3 can go on for years, but eventually the delay in insulin response causes blood-sugar levels to begin to peak above the normal range. The rollercoaster ride now becomes even wilder.

Two hours or so after a high carbohydrate meal, the blood-sugar level is higher than it should be, often provoking sleepiness.

Then the insulin level spikes, resulting in the symptoms of low blood sugar described above. This trio of conditions—insulin resistance, hyperinsulinism, and impaired glucose tolerance—is considered prediabetes.

Step 5: Type 2 Diabetes with Insulin Resistance and High Insulin Production

Eventually, although the pancreas continues to overproduce insulin, it no longer works in a timely fashion, resulting in dangerously high postprandial (after a meal) blood-sugar levels.

Step 6: Type 2 Diabetes with Little or No Insulin Production

Eventually, unless intervention occurs, the beta cells of the pancreas become dysfunctional and can no longer churn out insulin or produce inadequate amounts. In addition to elevated postprandial blood-sugar levels, fasting blood-sugar levels (at least eight hours after a meal) are also in the danger zone.

Often, only at this point, many people find out they have diabetes due to a host of symptoms that can include increased thirst, hunger, and need to urinate. Weight gain and blurred vision are other symptoms.

Indicators of Diabetes

Rather than relying on subjective symptoms, such as increase in thirst, we use the measurements of the metabolic syndrome to indicate diabetic conditions. The metabolic syndrome is a collection of five risk factors that dramatically increase the likelihood of developing type 2 diabetes, as well as coronary artery disease, stroke, hypertension, and Alzheimer's. Each of the five conditions is, in itself, a risk for diabetes and cardiovascular disease, but en masse, they vastly compound the likelihood of serious disease. You need have only three of these five conditions to be diagnosed with the metabolic syndrome:

- Truncal obesity. In men, this means a waist of forty inches or more; in women, thirty-five inches or more.

- Hypertension, meaning blood pressure of 135/85 mmHg or higher.

- High triglycerides, meaning 150 mg/dL or more.

- Low HDL ("good") cholesterol, meaning less than 40 mg/ dL for men and less than 50 mg/dL for women.

- High fasting blood sugar, meaning 110 mg/dL or higher.

Worldwide Proliferation of Diabetes

About 44 percent of Americans over the age of fifty have the metabolic syndrome, also known as prediabetes. According to the latest studies, there is no end in sight for the increasing rise in metabolic syndrome among Americans. As more and more people become overweight and obese, the hard numbers for metabolic syndrome rise at an alarming rate. In the United States, almost 21 million people, or 7 percent of the population, have diabetes, although almost one-third of them are unaware that they have the disease. Another 41 million have pre-diabetes.

Most children who have diabetes have type 1, which is the result of a lack of insulin, caused by the destruction of beta cells in the pancreas. Unfortunately, even children are demonstrating type 2 diabetes due to poor diet and inactivity. Type 2 diabetes in children is a growing concern. One-third of American children born in the year 2000 are predicted to develop type 2 diabetes.

The largest number of subjects showing metabolic syndrome are young women. And they are showing it at a younger and younger age.

Worldwide ballooning rates of type 2 diabetes have become an indictment of our lives of inactivity, overconsumption, as well as reliance on sweets and other junk foods full of empty carbohydrates. Even developing countries are seeing the incidence of diabetes skyrocket. China and India are now vying for the dubious distinction of having the largest number of diabetics in the world as economic growth and newfound prosperity has led to the adoption of Western eating habits and reduction in physical labor. In both societies, where malnutrition was long rampant, being plump and idle were traditionally seen as status symbols of affluence. Today, in both countries, obesity is fast becoming a public health issue among segments of the population.

Not far behind them, the United State is ranked third in the number of cases of diabetes in the world—and the top-ranked western/industrialized nation. The association of diabetes with affluence in developing countries, such as China and India, is in stark contrast with the United States, where diabetes is more common among the poor.

Here are some facts from the International Diabetes Federation.

- Type 2 diabetes affects more than 230 million people worldwide and is expected to affect 350 million by 2025.

- In 2003, the five countries with the largest numbers of people with diabetes were India (35.5 million), China (23.8 million), the United States (16 million), Russia (9.7 million), and Japan (6.7 million).

- By 2025, the number of people with diabetes is expected to more than double in Africa, the Eastern Mediterranean and Middle East, and Southeast Asia, and rise by 20 percent in Europe, 50 percent in North America, 85 percent in South and Central America, and 75 percent in the Western Pacific.

- Each year, a further 7 million people develop diabetes.

- Each year, over 3 million deaths are tied directly to diabetes. Every ten seconds, a person dies from diabetes-related causes.

- Diabetes is the fourth-leading cause of death by disease globally.

- At least 50 percent of all people with diabetes are unaware of their condition. In some countries, this figure may reach 80 percent.

The process that leads to type 2 diabetes can take years, but it does not necessarily proceed slowly. When you consider how most people eat and the fact that two-thirds of American adults are overweight or obese, it could seem that most of the population is likely to develop diabetes. Certainly the trend points in that direction. Researchers believe more fifty million Americans had metabolic syndrome in 1990. That number has skyrocketed to sixty-four million today and is beginning a geometric progression that will result in a huge number of Americans with heart disease and cognitive disorders in their old age.

Terrible as these statistics are, diabetes is also intimately linked to a number of other serious or life-threatening conditions, including heart disease, stroke, high blood pressure, kidney disease, blindness, amputations of digits or limbs, diseases of the nervous system, gum disease, sexual dysfunction and complications of pregnancy, and ultimately, Alzheimer's.

People with diabetes are two to four times more likely to develop cardiovascular disease (CVD) than people without diabetes. Cardiovascular disease is the number-one cause of death in industrialized countries. It is also set to overtake infectious diseases as the most common cause of death in many parts of the developing world. For each risk factor present, the risk of cardiovascular death is about three times greater in people with diabetes as compared to people without the condition.

Can this trend be stopped and even reversed?

We at the Salerno Center believe so. There is hope.

PREVENTING AND TREATING TYPE 2 DIABETES

Although the increasing number of people developing diabetes indicates a dire situation, it is not quite that bad. Some people have a built-in propensity to blood-sugar and insulin imbalances, and others do not. If you have such a propensity and never trigger it with overeating and eating the wrong kind of food, you may never know you have such an inclination.

However, for those who do show signs of sensitivity to insulin imbalances, we see the increasing incidence of diabetes as an opportunity to help people understand why low-carb diets, taken on at an early age, can prevent the deadly slide from metabolic syndrome to diabetes type 2, heart disease, Alzheimer's, and dementia.

Prospectively, an individual can handle this problem quite easily. For prevention and treatment of Alzheimer's and dementia, we teach people to eat a diet high in saturated fats and proteins from grass-fed meats and wild caught fish. We show them why they must avoid sugars and processed carbs of all kinds. Add exercise to the mix, and your chances for suffering this long slide into senility is greatly reduced. We have a long list of patients on our roster who are doing much better on this regimen.

Counterintuitive for many people, the results of our studies clearly demonstrate that eating saturated fat does not make you fat and does not lead to the dreaded metabolic syndrome.

Eating processed carbohydrates does.

Laboratory studies of blood samples shows that subjects who eat a low-fat diet, which is always high-carb, actually have worse fats in their bloodstream than those who eat a low-carb, high dietary-fat diet. We know from experience that not only do people lose weight but also their overall health improves on our low-carb regimen. Keeping blood glucose and insulin under control bodes well for a long and healthy life.

Case History

The Salerno Center has records of hundreds of patients who have used the Fight Fat with Fat Diet to treat type 2 diabetes and improve their health, often making dramatic improvements. Here is a typical case.

Mrs. T came to my center suffering from moderate obesity and type 2 diabetes. She was taking nearly one hundred units of insulin and was on Glucophage, a drug used to lower glucose levels. She was having difficulty losing weight, her blood sugars still averaged around 170, and she was tired all of the time and depressed. She was only forty-eight years old.

When she first came to the Salerno Center, we took extensive blood tests. In addition, after a fasting and two hours after eating a high-carb meal, insulin and glucose were taken. Mrs. T's insulin levels were through the roof, as were her glucose levels. Her thyroid gland was underactive, she had a huge amount of candida in her blood, and her triglycerides were extremely elevated, so typical for diabetics. Her blood pressure was also high. This poor women was a stroke or heart attack waiting to happen.

I placed Mrs. T immediately on a low carb, yeast-free diet where most cheeses, vinegar, and mushrooms were eliminated. She was placed on Salerno Glucose Factor, Salerno Multi vitamin, Anti-aging Factor, probiotic for yeast, and Salerno Blood Pressure Factor to lower her elevated blood pressure. She was also given a good amount of fish oils to lower her triglyceride level. Triglyceride elevation is much more problematic for stroke and heart disease, especially in women, than cholesterol levels. The fish oils were also given to decrease her blood thickness, which was also found to be elevated.

She was also placed on a thyroid medication. Her insulin injections were reduced to accommodate her new diet and vitamins. After one week, Mrs. T lost four pounds, and her insulin requirement decreased another 15 percent. Already, Mrs. T was feeling more energetic and less depressed. She lost another four pounds the following week and continued to reduce her insulin to nearly one-quarter of what she had begun with. By week sixteen, Mrs. T was completely off her insulin and had lost thirty-six pounds. She had not felt this great in years and had begun a running program. Mrs. T's triglycerides had normalized, her blood pressure was perfect, and by week forty-eight, she was even off her Glucophage medication.

Reducing Your Risk

The alarming epidemic in our country of type 2 diabetes is one malady that can be linked inextricably to our Western diet and life of inactivity and, thus, is almost completely preventable, provided you take a proactive stance against it. A modified version of the Fight Fat with Fat Diet and supplementation program could cut the risk of type 2 diabetes by over 95 percent in the general population.

The following strategies will help reduce your risks for type 2 diabetes.

- Know whether you have a family history of the disease.

- Lose weight if you are overweight (a BMI of more than 24.9).
- Exercise for a minimum of half an hour most days of the week.
- Do not drink alcohol in excess or at all if you have problems with unbalanced blood sugar.
- Obtain most of your carbohydrates from fresh, organic vegetables and some fruit and whole grains.
- Supplement your diet with recommended nutrients.
- After age forty-five, have your blood-sugar levels checked at least every three years.

Assessing Your Risks

A family history of diabetes is a clear message that you face an increased risk for the disease, along with several other matters beyond your control, but many critical factors are in your hands.

Age, Gender, and Race

Although type 2 diabetes increasingly strikes children and young adults, it is far more common in older people, particularly after age forty-five. Almost 21 percent of Americans aged sixty and older have diabetes.

Men are slightly more likely than women to get the disease, although African-American, Hispanic, Native American, Asian American, and Pacific Islander women are at least two to four times more likely than non-Hispanic white women to develop it.

Black Americans who do not have a Hispanic background are 1.8 times more likely to have diabetes than non-Hispanic whites. The same figure applies to residents of Puerto Rico. Mexican Americans are not far behind, being 1.7 times more at risk than non-Hispanic whites. Native Americans fare even worse—2.2 times more likely than non-Hispanic whites. Adult Hawaiians, whether natives or of Asian or Pacific island descent, are more than twice as likely to have diabetes than whites. Asian Americans living in California are at slightly less risk: 1.5 times that of non-Hispanic whites.

Surplus Pounds

I know I sound like a broken record, but as with numerous other diseases, being overweight increases the odds of developing diabetes. Being overweight—meaning a BMI above 24.9—is the biggest risk factor for type 2. When overweight gives way to obesity—meaning a BMI of 30 or more—the risk rises exponentially.

The younger a woman is when she puts on extra pounds, the more likely she will wind up as a diabetic. On the flip side, when women lose weight and keep it off, they can reduce their risk.

As with cardiovascular disease, where a person carries weight is significant. Apple-shaped men and women, who have thick waists—what doctors call truncal obesity—are more prone to diabetes than pear-shaped folks, who are heavy in the hips and buttocks.

For Women Only

Two conditions associated with the female reproductive system are also linked to the development of diabetes. If a woman has had what is called gestational diabetes during pregnancy (it goes away after she gives birth) or has given birth to an infant who weighed more than nine pounds, she has a greater likelihood of later developing type 2 diabetes.

Likewise, women with polycystic ovary syndrome (PCOS) have an elevated risk. PCOS is a hormonal imbalance associated with insulin resistance and high levels of insulin in the blood—similar to the early stages of diabetes—that afflicts up to 10 percent of all women in their childbearing years. It results in enlarged ovaries, irregular menstrual periods, failure to ovulate, weight gain, infertility, and excessive body hair due to excessive testosterone levels. About 35 percent of women with PCOS develop diabetes, and typically the disease progresses much more quickly than it does in women without PCOS.

In my practice, I have seen a low-carbohydrate-diet protocol will often lead to increased fertility.

The Danger of Inactivity

Although one can be overweight and still be physically active, inactivity is often a contributing factor to being overweight or obese. Exercise not only helps you maintain your healthy weight or weight loss; it also increases the ratio of muscle to fat in your body.

The more muscle mass you have, the higher your metabolism, which helps you burn more glucose and body fat. Also important, the more muscle you have, the more responsive your body is to the effects of insulin.

In fact, a review of fourteen studies has shown that even without significant weight loss, moderate exercise alone improves blood sugar control. Regular vigorous exercise works on multiple levels to reduce your risk for developing diabetes.

The Role of the Environment

A significant body of research links two toxins—arsenic and dioxins—to increased risk for diabetes.

Arsenic Assault

Although arsenic is present in the environment in many forms, the primary way in which the public is exposed to this poison is through contaminated drinking water and pesticides.

People are also exposed to arsenic in medicines to treat conditions as diverse as psoriasis and leukemia, as well as in some wines (likely via arsenic-laced pesticides) and mineral waters. Individuals who work in certain occupations, such as processing metal ores, manufacturing glass and pharmaceuticals, and producing or applying pesticides, are at heightened risk. Several research studies have shown an association between exposure to arsenic and increased risk of developing diabetes.

Deadly Dioxin

The term dioxin includes a family of highly persistent fat-soluble compounds found most commonly in foods high on the food chain, such as meat and dairy products. The most toxic form of dioxin is a byproduct of manufacturing and processing industries that use chlorine compounds. These include paper pulp mills, water and waste processors, and manufacturers of pesticides and polyvinyl chloride products. Dioxins also are spewed into the environment when chlorinated wastes are incinerated. In addition to a long list of health effects resulting from exposure to dioxins, high concentrations may alter glucose metabolism and hormonal levels.

Although the results of research have not been consistent, several findings suggest that dioxin exposure raises the risks for developing diabetes. Research on men who were involved in aerial spraying of herbicides, including Agent Orange, were more likely to have diabetes, impaired glucose metabolism, and impaired insulin production.

THE IMPORTANCE OF DIET

First of all, let me repeat:

**You can prevent diabetes from ever developing
by eating properly.**

Even if you already have disturbed blood-sugar and insulin resistance, you can stop them in their tracks without drugs, simply by changing the way you eat. This applies even if your parents and/ or siblings have type 2 diabetes.

The way of eating I advocate is not what the American Diabetic Association (ADA) recommends. Rather, instead of obsessing about fat and allowing plenty of sugar, white flour, and other nutritionally deficient foods, as the ADA program does, my approach comes from practices that bring verifiable and significantly positive results. People on the Fight Fat with Fat Diet lose weight, keep it off, and reduce or eliminate factors contributing to diabetes.

My work is derived from the work of Dr. Robert C. Atkins. Although his low-carbohydrate diet is best known for its weight-loss results, it is also key to avoiding diabetes. His program called for avoiding processed carbohydrates and eating only fiber- and nutrient-rich carbohydrates in combination with a mix of protein sources and natural fats. This diet makes it easy to keep weight under control. At the same time, it is ideally suited to managing blood sugar and insulin levels.

In fact, at the time of his death, Dr. Atkins was at work on the book he felt was the culmination of this life's work. *Atkins Diabetes Revolution: The Groundbreaking Approach to Preventing and Controlling Type 2 Diabetes* was published posthumously. Much of the book is based upon his observations working with thousands of patients, some of whom have since become my patients, who were able to correct their metabolic disorders by changing their diet, becoming physically active, and following a supplement protocol similar to the one I will describe later in this chapter.

This book is, of course, about prevention, so my focus is on how carbohydrate control effectively prevents diabetes.

Why Low Fat Does Not Work

Everyone agrees that keeping weight down reduces the risk of getting diabetes, as well as heart disease and a host of other conditions discussed in this book.

Long term, the best way to control your weight is to develop healthful eating habits and eat moderately. Do that, and unless you have a major metabolic disorder and are extremely inactive, you will arrive at a weight that is appropriate for your age and body type.

But if a diet—and I am speaking of a way of eating, not specifically a weight-loss diet—is impossible to maintain because it is lacking in flavor and leaves you hungry and with cravings for certain foods, it is only a matter of time before it becomes a former diet. In the decades since the American government has advocated a low-fat diet, the obesity epidemic has exploded.

Low Fat Is High Carb

A low-fat diet, by definition, is inherently a high-carbohydrate diet. That is because when you restrict fat you are restricting protein as well since meat, poultry, fish, cheese, and most other forms of protein contain good amounts of fat. What you are left with, then, is carbohydrates, which encompasses an array of foods. (Most foods contain some combination of fat, protein, and carbohydrate.) Low-glycemic ("good") carbohydrates are typically whole foods, like leafy green vegetables, brown rice, lentils, raspberries, and hundreds of other vegetables, fruits, and whole grains.

Then there is the endless array of high-glycemic ("bad") carbohydrates that beckon from the supermarket shelves, including the processed, refined offerings, such as cookies, chips, syrupy drinks, white bread, and so on. By definition, high glycemic foods have a dramatic impact on blood sugar levels within a couple of hours after consumption.

In contrast, low glycemic foods raise blood-sugar levels more slowly and moderately. In addition, dairy products contain carbohydrate, along with fat and protein.

Carbs, Blood Sugar, and Insulin

While it is definitely possible to eat a high carbohydrate diet comprised primarily of fresh vegetables, whole grains, and fruits—witness the Mediterranean cuisine—with a modest amount of fish, cheese, and meat, in this country, a so-called low-fat diet is usually packed with high-glycemic carbohydrates. And for someone with a genetic propensity to diabetes, that is a recipe for disaster.

Here is why.

When you indulge in high-glycemic, refined-carbohydrate foods, your blood sugar quickly rises prompting your pancreas to release insulin to ferry the blood sugar to your cells. If you continue to eat this way, over time, the cells become increasingly resistant to the effects of the insulin, stimulating the pancreas to produce even more insulin.

When the insulin finally does the trick, your blood-sugar level dips so low that it can stimulate stress hormones that cause hunger and cravings for sweets and other carbohydrate foods. When you give into those cravings, the cycle repeats itself, and the pounds pile on.

It is these cravings that distinguish the condition known as carbohydrate addiction, which makes it so difficult for some people to take control of their weight. In addition to prompting the storage of excess glucose as body fat, the release of insulin has another dangerous result. The fat is transported around your body in the bloodstream in the form of triglycerides. High triglycerides, you will recall, are an independent risk factor for diabetes.

Most Fats Are Fine

When you control carbohydrates, you do not have to keep track of your consumption of fat—other than trans fats, known as hydrogenated or partially hydrogenated oils, which are to be avoided at all costs.

That means that you can enjoy a lamb chop, salmon, olive oil on your vegetables and in your salad dressing, and whipped cream on fresh raspberries without feeling guilty. In fact, all of these fats carry flavor, which makes food more satisfying.

When you eliminate most fat from your diet, you yearn for flavor, which can often lead to overeating. Fats provide a comforting satiety in a way that carbohydrates do not.

CONQUERING SYSTEMIC YEAST INFECTIONS

Defining Systemic Yeast

Systemic yeast, or *Candida albicans*, is a fungal organism that is present in everyone's intestinal tract. It is normally kept under control by the immune system and by beneficial intestinal bacteria. This balance is upset when these bacteria are destroyed (often by antibiotics), when our immune function is impaired by stress or illness, or when we develop environmental or food sensitivities. Then, *Candida* begins to proliferate and invade and colonize our body tissues. It most commonly appears as a vaginal yeast infection or as oral thrush. But *Candida albicans* can also spread inside the body and become a systemic problem.

Case History

Amy came to my office by referral from another diet doctor. She had been on a low-carb diet, but her weight loss had stalled out, and she was feeling depressed and had been craving sugar.

Her other symptoms included diarrhea, bloating, gas, fatigue, insomnia, and frequent lower abdominal pain, especially after eating. She had seen a succession of doctors, including a gastroenterologist, who told her she had irritable bowel syndrome (IBS) and recommended a high-fiber diet.

Like many women with similar problems, Amy had tried several regimens without success. She had started out well in a weight-loss program, but it had stalled out, and she still had about forty-five pounds to lose. With the added problems of sugar cravings, fatigue, bloating, and pain, she had about given up. She was really feeling bad.

I believed that Amy was suffering from systemic yeast, or *Candida*, often accompanied by dysbiosis, which is an imbalance of the bacteria in the intestines. Parasites, yeast overgrowth, high-sugar content, and food allergies, all can cause dysbiosis. And all of this causes weight gain.

While I was taking her history, Amy reported she had been on vacation in Mexico in the spring and that had been the end of success with her diet. I knew it was also probably the beginning of her problems with yeast and parasites.

We did a conventional work-up on her, including a stool test, which did, indeed, reveal the presence of parasites, systemic yeast, and imbalanced bacterial flora—the true underlying causes of her symptoms and the reason her diet was no longer working.

The parasites were the easy part. The systemic yeast was the more difficult problem. But when she adhered to the Fight Fat with Fat Diet, along with supplements, and some IV vitamins, she conquered her systemic yeast, and she lost the weight.

How *Candida Albicans* Affects the Body

When *Candida* proliferates, it changes from its simple, relatively harmless form to an invasive form, with long root-like structures that penetrate the intestinal lining. Penetration can break down the boundary between the intestinal tract and the circulatory system. This may allow into the bloodstream many substances, which may be systemic allergens, poisons, or irritants. Partially digested proteins may enter the blood through the openings created by *Candida* (called leaky-gut syndrome), which explains why individuals with *Candida* also often display a variety of food and environmental allergies.

Symptoms of *Candida* Yeast Infections

While many of these symptoms may be caused by conditions other than candidiasis, a woman suffering from systemic yeast will typically experience various symptoms in a number of areas.

- Weight: If she has been on a diet, it will no longer work. If she has not been on a diet, she may experience an unexplained weight gain.

- Generalized: Fatigue, lethargy, migraine headaches, weakness, dizziness, sensory disturbances, hypoglycemia, muscle pain, respiratory problems, chemical sensitivities.

- Gastrointestinal: Oral thrush, diarrhea, constipation, rectal itching, inflammatory bowel disease (IBD), flatulence, food sensitivities.

- Genitourinary: Yeast vaginitis, menstrual and premenstrual problems, bladder inflammation, chronic urinary tract infections (UTIs), bladder inflammation, cystitis, PMS.

- Dermatological: Eczema, acne, hives.

- Mental and emotional: Panic attacks, confusion, irritability, memory loss, inability to concentrate, depression, insomnia, learning disability, short attention span.

- Autoimmune: Multiple sclerosis, arthritis, systemic lupus erythematosus, myasthenia gravis, scleroderma, hemolytic anemia, sarcoidosis, thrombocytopenic purpura.

Diagnosis of Systemic Yeast (*Candida*) Infection

A simple stool test can determine if someone has *Candida* yeast overgrowth.

Treatment of Systemic Yeast (*Candida*) Infection

We recommend dietary changes, supplements, and lifestyle changes that provide a natural remedy for candidiasis. The Fight Fat with Fat Diet is a good basic diet to follow to rid yourself of a systemic yeast problem. The diet is high in whole foods with plenty of vegetables, protein, and natural fat and has virtually no simple sugars, processed carbohydrates, or artificial colors, sweeteners, and dyes.

Foods to avoid in a *Candida* diet

1. Avoid yeast-containing foods

- Beer, wine, and all other forms of alcohol
- Breads, rolls, pretzels, pastries, cookies, and sweet rolls
- B-complex vitamins and selenium products, unless labeled "yeast-free"
- Vinegar or foods containing vinegar, such as mustard, salad dressings, pickles, barbeque sauce, mayonnaise
- Commercially prepared foods, such as soups, dry roasted nuts, potato chips, soy sauce, cider, natural root beer, olives, sauerkraut

2. Avoid mold-containing and mold-supporting foods

- Pickled, smoked, or dried meats, fish, and poultry
- Cured pork bacon
- All cheese, aged or fresh, except cream cheese and fresh mozzarella

- Mushrooms
- Tempeh
- Soy sauce, tamari, and miso
- Peanuts, peanut products, and pistachios
- Herbs and teas that may be moldy
- Malt or foods containing malt
- Canned or prepared tomatoes (fresh tomatoes are fine)

3. Avoid all sugars

- Honey, maple syrup, brown sugar
- Fruit juices (canned, bottled, or frozen)
- Dried fruits
- All processed sugar
- Anything containing high-fructose corn syrup
- High glycemic index foods
- All prepared and processed foods for a period of at least four weeks
- All alcohol

Foods you can eat in a *Candida* diet

- All fresh non-starchy vegetables—a large variety, raw, steamed, or sautéed in butter or olive oil—including plenty of dark green leafy vegetables
- Fresh protein at every meal, including beef, chicken, fish, turkey, eggs, and shellfish. Organic is best, but fresh is essential. Choose grass-fed meats and wild-caught fish.
- Unprocessed nuts and seeds, except peanuts.
- Unrefined cold-pressed olive, sesame, and coconut oils.

- Lemon juice with oil for salad dressing. This may be a prepared product, but be careful to avoid any salad dressing that contains vinegar.

- Beverages such as mineral or spring water, coffee, and tea.

- Limited quantities of low-sugar, fresh fruit (three daily), unless you see a reaction; then limit to twice weekly.

Most often, we recommend the patient stay on this program for four months and then repeat the stool test. In that time, the patient has usually made enough progress to wean off the anti-fungal agent and the probiotic supplement and to moderate the anti-yeast diet.

In our personal program, we provide pharmaceutical-grade supplements plus optional phone support from our Nurse-Educators. While the personal program is not a medical practice, many women find the right combination of guidance and support from our nurses, who are highly trained.

REGULATING BLOOD-SUGAR LEVELS

One of the most persistent problems that my patients tell me about when they come in for their first visit is a lack of energy, sometimes followed by explosive bursts of temper, foggy thinking, and other unpleasant effects from eating a diet high in sugars and carbohydrates. These people did not come to me to correct their low energy or quick temper, and often they do not even know there is a connection between the way they feel and what they eat. But the connection is clear. These patients are on a daily fun-house ride that seems painfully slow at times and explosively fast at others.

In medicine, we know this to be the result of fluctuating blood sugars. You eat pancakes for breakfast with syrup, and you feel like a million until about 10 a.m. when, all of a sudden, you find yourself sweaty, cranky, irritable, and sometimes even faint. So what do you do? Grab a donut and a cup of coffee? I hope not, but that is often the answer. Then the fun house starts all over again, ultimately plunging you into a dark, scary place, and you feel as if you will never get out.

What most of these patients came to see me about is overweight and obesity. Many of them have tried punishing diets with almost no protein or fat, often vegetarian, and with such low calories that their body is thrown into a tantrum of fluctuating blood sugars.

The Dangers of Blood Sugar Fluctuation

A low level of blood sugar, referred to as hypoglycemia, results in an inadequate supply of glucose to the brain. Hypoglycemia can cause a number unpleasant symptoms, including fatigue, weakness, dizziness, inability to concentrate, poor memory, anxiety, depression, irritability, heart palpitations, and excessive sweating. It can even cause comas and seizures.

On the other end of the spectrum, a high level of blood sugar is referred to as hyperglycemia and is one of the key symptoms of diabetes. Hyperglycemia can cause similar symptoms to hypoglycemia, such as fatigue, inability to concentrate, anxiety, and depression. However, it can also cause shortness of breath, nausea, dry mouth, and in severe cases, even comas, nerve damage, and blindness.

Blood-sugar fluctuation puts a significant demand on the glands responsible for regulating it, and this burden is one of the major reasons that fluctuating blood sugar is such a serious health concern. It is widely recognized as the cause of type 2 diabetes and is also associated with high blood pressure and heart disease.

How the Body Responds to Blood Sugar Fluctuation

High levels of blood sugar trigger the pancreas to respond in emergency-like fashion by quickly releasing a large amount of insulin. By facilitating the transport of blood glucose into cells and the conversion of excess blood glucose into body fat, the presence of insulin causes blood sugar to drop.

However, the large amount of insulin often causes too much glucose to be removed from the blood and results in a state of hypoglycemia. The excessive drop in blood sugar creates another state of emergency and stimulates the adrenal glands to release cortisol. This increases blood sugar to a desirable level by facilitating the creation of glucose from body fat and muscle tissue and also by stimulating the liver to create glucose from its storage of glycogen.

While the mechanisms involved in blood sugar regulation provide us with an invaluable source of protection, they also put a significant physiological burden on the body. The continuous demand put on the pancreas to produce excessive amounts of insulin eventually leads to type 2 diabetes. In similar fashion, the recurring need for the adrenal glands to produce cortisol can compromise their capacity as well and result in adrenal fatigue. Although adrenal fatigue is not as widely recognized as diabetes, it can be equally problematic and result in susceptibility to significant health problems. Furthermore, any type of adrenal stimulation, including low blood sugar, invokes the universal stress response that is so frequently associated with poor health.

Tips for Regulating Blood Sugar

One of the best things you can do for your health is to keep your blood sugar at a relatively consistent level. The following tips will help to spare your body from the significant burden of blood-sugar fluctuation and will help you maintain a steady mood and energy level while making your weight-loss program both possible and pleasant.

- Choose the Fight Fat with Fat Diet as your bible. This will give you a step-by-step instruction for regulating your blood sugars while you lose weight.

- Eliminate sugar and refined carbohydrates from your diet, or keep them to an absolute minimum. If you have any excess body fat, eliminating these foods will help you lose weight in addition to keeping your blood sugar stabilized.

- Minimize your intake of caffeine. Drink lemon water instead.

- Follow a consistent eating schedule with five small meals a day, and try not to go more than four hours without a meal.

- Some fruits and vegetables can cause blood sugar fluctuation just as easily as processed foods. See the sections, "Foods to Adore" and "Foods to Abhor" in Part III: The Fight Fat with Fat Marathon, for a list of specific fruits and vegetable to enjoy or to avoid.

Remember, you can control your blood-sugar level through the action you take—or fail to take. The Fight Fat with Fat Diet, detailed later in this book, will guide you in keeping your blood sugar at a safe and even level, as well as maintaining a healthy weight and lifestyle.

BIO-IDENTICAL HORMONE REPLACEMENT THERAPY

Bio-identical Hormone Replacement Therapy Defined

Bio-identical hormone replacement therapy, or BHRT, treats the symptoms of menopause, perimenopause, and postmenopause. Those symptoms can include hot flashes, bloating, weight gain, mood swings, and brain fog.

BHRT and Chronic Fatigue Syndrome

By its very nature, chronic fatigue depletes the body's natural hormones. It is important to understand chronic fatigue as a self-cycling, downward spiral that must be interrupted by a careful diagnosis, then a regimen of bio-identical hormones, natural thyroid replacement, and a well-thought out all-natural diet of unprocessed foods, as well as help optimizing sleep and rest.

In my practice, I often find chronic-fatigue patients deficient in hormones. Replacing them as naturally as possible is the best way to balance the body so the patient can quickly experience symptom relief. These hormones include estrogen, progesterone, testosterone, DHEA, and pregnenolone.

Role of Bio-identical Hormone Treatments in Fatigued Patients

Balancing the hormone deficiency with bio-identical hormones when combined with diet and support will increase strength, stamina, mood, and motivation. We run a comprehensive blood test to determine the exact combination of bio-identical hormones that will best balance each patient's body.

Thyroid health is also an important factor. To get a more in-depth view of how the patient's thyroid is working, we do a special test, the Thyroid Releasing Hormone Stimulation test (TRH). The TRH test is different from the more common TSH (thyroid stimulating hormone) test and sometimes catches imbalances that the TSH test cannot.

Making sure the thyroid is functioning properly is essential for total wellness and relief from fatigue. We prescribe a natural thyroid replacement, which is much more effective than the synthetic treatment often suggested.

Diet and Nutrition in Chronic Fatigue Syndrome

A well-balanced diet of organic, unprocessed foods with sufficient protein and natural fats is most beneficial to the chronic-fatigue patient.

A poor diet is one of the most important factors that contribute to fatigue. This life-changing plan is beneficial to the chronic fatigue syndrome, or CFS, patient as well as to people who wish to normalize their weight and increase their stamina and general health to look forward to a long and vigorous life.

I have had great success with CFS patients by combining the Fight Fat with Fat Diet with a regimen of bio-identical hormones, thyroid, and recommendations for improved sleep and exercise.

Specific Food Recommendations for CFS

I highly recommend a low carb diet of unprocessed and organic foods to improve CFS symptoms.

Avoid completely or have only a very few refined carbohydrates or processed foods. It is so easy and yet so hard for most Americans to realize how important it is to eliminate all processed foods, sugars and bad carbs, such as highly refined carbohydrates in store-bought breads, cookies, chips, crackers, and other snack foods that are packaged or boxed.

The diet MUST consist of organic food as much as possible. Focus on wild-caught fish, organic vegetables, grass-fed meats, organic eggs, and full-fat cheeses, which are all well tolerated by the CFS patient. Add dark-colored fruits, including berries, which are also recommended. Eating whole, unprocessed organic foods helps the body's natural functions to be optimized, excess weight is lost, and overall health is restored. I recommend not only a special diet for the CFS patient but also a plan to improve the health of every member of the family.

Caffeine in moderation, generally, is acceptable as it can increase energy. Overuse of caffeine or any stimulant, including sugar and all its derivatives, can make it difficult to fall asleep and stay asleep. Getting plenty of rest is imperative in allowing the body to heal and to stay in balance. Consume NO coffee or caffeine-laced products (including chocolate) after the afternoon.

Stimulants and ADHD Drugs

Stimulants and ADHD drugs must be avoided as they will cause long-term issues and eventually serious side effects, which can, if untreated, be fatal. Some good alternatives to these stimulants are all-natural supplements that can replace what is most deficient in the body. Supplements such as L-Carnatine, Coenzyme Q-10, D-Ribose, B12, and L-Taurine work very nicely and have no side effects.

THE IMPORTANCE OF SUPPLEMENTS

A good program of supplements acts as an insurance policy, even when you follow a healthful diet. The following supplements promote the metabolism of carbohydrates, improve insulin sensitivity, lower triglycerides, and act as anti-inflammatories.

Alpha Lipoic Acid

The antioxidant alpha lipoic acid assists the body in using glucose, which enables it to improve blood-sugar control. In one study, people with type 2 diabetes who were give intravenous supplemental alpha lipoic acid (ALA) saw an increase in insulin release and a reduction in blood sugar levels.

One way in which antioxidants, of which ALA is one, help fight diabetes is by neutralizing free radicals in your body involved in the development of insulin resistance. Supplementing with ALA has been shown to enhance uptake of glucose by tissues.

One serious complication of diabetes is nerve damage, called diabetic neuropathy, which results in pain, tingling, and numbness in the extremities. It can be relieved with supplemental ALA. One study (see http://www.ncbi.nlm.nih.gov/pubmed/7587852) showed that nerve function was restored after four months on high oral doses. "Alpha lipoic acid improves nerve blood flow, reduces oxidative stress, and improves distal nerve conduction in experimental diabetic neuropathy."

Optimal daily dose: 600–1000 mg alpha lipoic acid.

Banaba Leaf Extract

Long used in the Philippines as a natural plant insulin for blood sugar control, banaba leaf appears to balance blood sugar by promoting healthy insulin levels and stimulating the transport of glucose into cells. It also is said to help control cravings, particularly for carbohydrates, and may promote weight loss.

In a clinical study of people with type 2 diabetes who received a standardized extract of banaba leaf that contained 1 percent corosolic acids showed a 30 percent decrease in blood sugar levels after two weeks.

Optimal daily dose: 50 mg banaba leaf extract.

Biotin

A water-soluble B vitamin, also known as vitamin H, biotin is key to the metabolism of energy, enabling four essential enzymes to break down carbohydrates into glucose, fats into fatty acids, and protein into amino acids.

Produced in the body by certain types of intestinal bacteria, biotin is also found in foods, such as brewer's yeast, nutritional yeast, oat bran, whole grains, nuts and nut butters, egg yolks, sardines, legumes, liver and other organ meats, bananas, cauliflower, and mushrooms.

People with type 2 diabetes often are deficient in biotin. Long-term use of antibiotics can also depress levels.

Optimal daily dose: 2–4 mg biotin.

Note: Biotin appears to work synergistically with chromium to control blood sugar, so be sure to take the two supplements together.

Chromium

Like biotin, the trace mineral chromium plays a role in the metabolism of carbohydrates, protein, and fat, helping your body metabolize fat, turn protein into muscle, and convert carbohydrate into energy. Chromium used to be abundant in the soil, but industrial farming and the overuse of pesticides and herbicides have leached the soils of most of this vital nutrient.

Chromium is necessary to make glucose tolerance factor, which enhances the action of insulin, facilitating the process by which glucose is transported to the liver, muscle, and fat cells, where it can be converted into energy as needed, thereby keeping blood sugar levels under control.

Deficiency in chromium results in impaired glucose tolerance, insulin resistance, and diabetes-like symptoms. In addition, chromium acts as an appetite suppressant.

Chromium supplements have also been shown to improve glucose tolerance and reduce abnormally high blood levels of insulin in pregnant women with gestational diabetes. Since heart disease is often a complication of diabetes, improvements in cholesterol and triglycerides are valuable benefits.

Vigorous exercise can deplete the body's stores of chromium. Processing foods also depletes them of most of the trace mineral. Trace amounts of chromium are found in many foods, among them brewer's yeast, beef, cheese, leafy dark greens, mushrooms, shellfish, and barley.

Optimal daily dose: 200–600 mcg chromium.

Note: Chromium should be taken with biotin for maximum effectiveness.

Cinnamon Bark

Next time you sprinkle cinnamon on your cappuccino or your oatmeal, you may also be cutting your risk for diabetes and cardiovascular disease. The familiar spice is a potent antioxidant with the potential to help maintain healthy blood sugar and cholesterol levels. The Chinese used cinnamon for an array of medical complaints, ranging from diarrhea to influenza, as long as four thousand years ago.

It was also used, as many spices were, to preserve food in the days before refrigeration.

Regular supplementation with cinnamon may be able to reduce fasting blood sugar, triglycerides, LDL cholesterol, and total cholesterol. Supplementation does not improve glycemic control in postmenopausal women.

Optimal daily dose: 125–250 mg cinnamon bark.

Coenzyme Q-10

This micronutrient is produced by the body, but production slows with age. Coenzyme Q-10 plays an important role in producing energy for the mitochondria found in every cell in your body. People with diabetes typically have lower levels of Co-Q-10 than do healthy people.

Optimal daily dose: 100–300 mg Co-Q-10.

Gymnema Sylvestre

Also known as gurmar and meshasringa, the leaves of the plant gymnema sylvestre have been used for centuries in Ayurvedic medicine to regulate glucose metabolism. In fact, the Hindi name gurmar translates as "sugar destroyer."

Unlike a prescription drug, gymnema lowers blood sugar levels gradually by helping regenerate the beta cells in the pancreas that secrete insulin, thus raising insulin levels. Unlike insulin and other drugs, gymnema will not reduce blood sugar to dangerous levels.

It also interferes with glucose absorption in the intestine, which helps keep the pancreas from releasing too much insulin. The herb also helps the uptake of glucose by the cells and keeps adrenaline from stimulating the liver to produce glucose.

Finally, gymnema banishes the taste of sugar, which suppresses cravings for sweets, making it easier to lose weight.

Optimal daily dose: 500 mcg. gymnema sylvestre.

Magnesium

Magnesium lowers blood glucose levels, increases insulin sensitivity, and calms the sympathetic nervous system.

Although the relationship between magnesium and diabetes has been studied for decades, it is still poorly understood. However, what is known about diabetes and magnesium embodies a persuasive list encouraging supplementation.

Low magnesium levels are common findings in non-insulin-dependent diabetic patients. (Philip Domenico and James R. Komorowski, "Mineral and Insulin Health" in *Nutraceuticals, Glycemic Health and Type 2 Diabetes*, ed. Vijai K. Pasupuleti and James W. Anderson [New York: John Wiley & Sons, 2009], 179.) In fact, diabetes is a frequent cause of secondary hypomagnesemia (lower blood levels of magnesium). Poorly controlled diabetics excrete more magnesium than do non-diabetics.

Magnesium assists in the maintenance of functional beta cells (insulin factories). (Kowluru et al. 2001, http://www.lifeextensionvitamins.com/nuinforprand2.html) Scientists believe that a magnesium deficiency interrupts insulin secretion and its activity. Magnesium, by enhancing the action of insulin, improves insulin's ability to transport glucose into the cell.

Magnesium increases the number and sensitivity of insulin receptors. (Waterfall 2000, http://www.lifeextensionvitamins.com/nuinforprand2.html) Borth the references are on this website.

An increase in red blood cell magnesium, which assesses the overall status of magnesium in the body, significantly and positively correlated with an increase in both insulin secretion and action. Correction of low erythrocyte magnesium concentrations may allow for improved glucose handling, particularly in elderly diabetic patients (http://www.lifeextensionvitamins.com/nuin-forprand2.html).

As magnesium levels plummet, the incidence of diabetic complications escalates. Magnesium is the mineral of choice to reduce hyper-responsiveness occurring in the sympathetic nervous system (SNS). This is important to the diabetic because, when the SNS is alerted, blood glucose levels tend to be higher.

The SNS is also associated with fostering greater levels of stress and anxiety, earning its reputation as the "flight or fight" division. Since diabetes is considered to be a disease promulgated by stress, supplementation that favors an inner calm is of significant advantage.

**Optimal daily dose: 750 mg. magnesium,
divided into two doses.**

N-Acetyl-L-Cysteine

N-acetyl-L-cysteine (NAC) is a form of the amino acid cysteine, which helps the body synthesize the antioxidant glutathione that has been shown to improve insulin sensitivity. When insulin levels are high, free radicals flourish, which can destroy various types of tissue.

Optimal daily dose: 600–1200 mgs NAC.

Note: NAC should be accompanied by 15 mg of zinc and 2 mg of copper per day.

Resveratrol

Resveratrol is a polyphenol found in red wine and some plants and has antioxidant properties. In November 2008, researchers at the Weill Medical College of Cornell University reported that dietary supplementation with resveratrol significantly reduced plaque formation in animal brains, a component of Alzheimer's and other neurodegenerative diseases. In humans, it is theorized that oral doses of resveratrol may reduce beta amyloid plaque associated with aging changes in the brain. Researchers theorize that one mechanism for plaque eradication is the ability of resveratrol to chelate (bind) copper. The neuroprotective effects have been confirmed in several animal model studies.

The anti-inflammatory effects of resveratrol have been demonstrated in several animal model studies. Resveratrol has showed promise as a potential therapy for arthritis.

It has long been known that moderate drinking of red wine reduces the risk of heart disease. This is best known as "the French paradox." Studies suggest that resveratrol in red wine may play an important role in this phenomenon. The cardioprotective effects of resveratrol are also theorized to be a form of preconditioning—the best method of cardioprotection, rather than direct therapy.

Resveratrol ameliorates common diabetes symptoms, such as polyphagia, polydipsia, and body weight loss. In human clinical trials, resveratrol has lowered blood sugar levels in both Phase Ib and Phase IIa.

Studies show that resveratrol inhibits herpes simplex virus (HSV) types 1 and 2 replication by inhibition of an early step in the virus replication cycle.

Studies also show that resveratrol inhibits varicella-zoster virus, certain influenza virus, respiratory viruses, and human cytomegalovirus. Furthermore, resveratrol synergistically enhances the anti-HIV-1 activity of several anti-HIV drugs.

Optimal daily dose: 500 mgs resveratrol.

Vanadium

Along with biotin and chromium, vanadium helps get the proper amounts of glucose into the body's cells. This trace mineral is found in black pepper, mushrooms, sunflower and safflower seeds and oil, olive oil, shellfish, parsley, dill seed, buckwheat, oats, rice, green beans, carrots, cabbage, radishes, and eggs. In vivo and in vitro studies have shown that vanadium mimics the effects of insulin.

Vanadium can lower blood sugar levels and improve sensitivity to insulin in both type 1 and type 2 diabetes.

In parts of the world where industrial farming practices have not leached the soils of vanadium and selenium, there are lower-than-average rates of heart disease. Nonetheless, too much vanadium can be dangerous.

Optimal daily dose: 30–60 mg vanadyl sulfate or 1–2 mg vanadyl.

Note: Excessive levels of vanadyl can be toxic so take care not to exceed dosage.

PART II

THE FIGHT FAT WITH FAT DIET DETOX FULL FAT FAST

HOW TO START THE FIGHT FAT WITH FAT DIET

You will start the Fight Fat with Fat Diet with a short period of detoxification, the Full Fat Fast, specified in this section. The next chapter will provide you with information, including recipes, for the diet after this initial detoxification.

The Fight Fat with Fat Detox Full Fat Fast gives your body a rest from the assaults of the Western diet. Getting rid of carbs from your diet will quickly put your body into fat-burning mode, and if you adhere to this for two weeks, you will lose from five to fifteen pounds and two inches off your waist.

Here is a step-by-step guide to your day on the Fight Fat with Fat Detox Full Fat Fast. Make a copy and put this on your refrigerator for ready reference.

Fight Fat with Fat Detox Full Fat Fast

- Within one hour of rising each morning, eat two large organic eggs, cooked any way you like (suggestions and recipes below). You can add a side of bacon, sausage, or ham if you want, and you can also have coffee or tea with cream and non-sugar sweetener (such as stevia or Splenda). Make sure fat fast has 0 carbs, 0 fruit, and 0 vegetables.

- Three hours later, have a small snack: a stick of string cheese, a handful of nuts, jerky, an ounce of sausage, or even some pork skins. Add another cup of coffee or tea with cream and non-sugar sweetener if you wish.

- Eat lunch three hours later: two ounces of cooked steak, hamburger, lamb chop, pork chop, any preservative-free sausage, salmon, sardines with mustard, or tuna salad made with regular mayonnaise. You may even choose a couple more eggs, perhaps made into a salad.

- Three hours later have another snack of about fifteen nuts (macadamias, Brazils, walnuts, hazelnuts, pecans, or pistachios are fine). A handful of pork skins, a stick of cheese, or some jerky is also okay.

- Have dinner three hours later: another two ounces of steak, burger, chops, poultry, or fish.

- Drink lots of water-based liquids during the day, at least sixty-four ounces. Coffee with heavy cream is fine, iced tea with fresh mint, or lemon water, which is ice water with a squirt of lemon juice and a packet of sugar substitute. Stevia is best, but sucralose (Splenda) is fine too. Remember that these products are much sweeter than sugar, so use a small amount in the water. Plain, old-fashioned water is perhaps the best choice. Just drink and drink and drink.

- On the first day of your fast, measure yourself. Weigh in and write it down. Use a tape measure around your waist. After a week, weigh yourself again, and then one week later, weigh yourself one more time at the end of the Full Fat Fast.

- After three or four days, you may experience constipation. Correct with a daily serving of Miracle Noodles (www.MiracleNoodle.com) or shirataki at the Asian market nearest you. These all-fiber, no carb, no calorie foods from Asia are a life saver. See recipes at the Miracle Noodle site, or simply do what we do—rinse the noodles in boiling water, drain, put in ziplock bags, then around midafternoon, eat three tablespoons or so with a drop or two of your favorite no-carb salad dressing. You will never be hungry; you will never be constipated. This works.

FOODS TO ADORE	
Fats	Extra-virgin olive oil, butter, unrefined flax oil, fresh lard, foie gras, nuts (walnuts, pecans, Brazil nuts, and hazelnuts)
Proteins	Organic or grass-fed beef, pork, veal, lamb, game, chicken, turkey, duck and other fowl (where possible). Chicken or veal liver, nitrate-free bacon and sausage, all seafood from cold, deep water (including codfish, halibut, and salmon), shellfish, and eggs
Dairy	Butter, raw-milk cheeses, organic full-fat milk, yogurt, buttermilk, heavy and sour cream from pasture-fed cows
Beverages	At least 64 ounces a day of water, lemon water, coffee, tea
Condiments	Sea salt, best quality balsamic vinegar, apple cider vinegar, rice wine vinegar, mayonnaise, mustard, soy sauce, fish sauce

FOODS TO ABHOR	
Fats	Highly processed vegetable oils (such as canola or soybean), margarine, vegetable shortening
Proteins	Processed meats
Dairy	Processed cheeses, reduced or non-fat dairy products
Carbohydrates	For the detox phase, avoid starchy fruits and foods made from white flour (including bread, cookies, crackers, pastas, and dry cereals), high fructose corn syrups, refined sugars, irradiated or genetically modified grains, chocolate mixed with sugar in any form
Beverages	Soda (including diet or sugar free), all fruit juices, beer, wine, rice milk, soy milk
Condiments	Catsup, commercial baking powder, MSG, artificial flavors, artificial additives, and artificial colors

DETOX RECIPES AND MENU SUGGESTIONS

Eggs, your new best friend

Eggs contain the highest quality of protein available and almost every essential vitamin and mineral needed by humans, which is why in the Full Fat Fast you will be eating two every morning for breakfast. In fact, egg protein is of such high quality that it is used as the standard by which other proteins are compared.

Eggs have a biological value (efficacy with which protein is used for growth) of 93.7%. Comparable values are 84.5% for milk, 76% for fish, and 74.3% for beef. Eggs really are the best protein money can buy, and it has all of those other valuable vitamins and minerals too.

Nutritional Content of a Large Egg			
Nutrient (unit)	Whole Egg	Egg White	Egg Yolk
Calories (kcal)	72	17	53
Protein (g)	6.28	3.64	2.63
Carbohydrate (g)	.36	.60	.24
Total Fat (g)	4.76	0.06	4.41
Saturated Fat (g)	1.6	0.0	1.6

Nutritional Content of a Large Egg			
Monosaturated fat (g)	1.9	0.0	1.9
Polysaturated fat (g)	1.0	0.0	0.7
Cholesterol (mg)	186	0	180
Thiamin (mg)	0.020	Trace	0.029
Riboflavin (mg)	0.229	0.088	0.147
Folate (mcg)	24	1	24
Vitamin B6 (mg)	0.085	0.002	0.058
Vitamin B12 (mcg)	0.45	0.32	0.03
Vitamin A (IU)	270	0.00	239
Vitamin E (mg)	0.53	0.00	0.43
Vitamin D (IU)	41	0.0	36
Choline (mg)	146.9	0.4	136.2
Calcium (mg)	28	2	21
Iron (mg)	0.88	.03	0.45
Magnesium (mg)	6	4	1
Copper (mg)	0.036	0.013	0.008
Zinc (mg)	0.65	0.01	0.38
Sodium (mg)	71	55	8
Potassium (mg)	69	54	18
Phosphorus (mg)	99	5	65
Lutein & Zeaxanthin (mcg)	166.5	0.0	186

Source: USDA National Nutrient Database (2012).

Eggs have long been an important contributor to the nutritional quality of the American diet. As the following chart from the USDA demonstrates, eggs supply a higher percentage of many nutrients to the diet than food energy, or calories.

Nutrient	Percentage (%)
Food Energy	1.3
Protein	3.9
Fat	2.0
Vitamin A	4.3
Vitamin E	4.3
Riboflavin	6.4
Vitamin B6	2.1
Vitamin B12	3.7
Folate	5.1
Iron	2.4
Phosphorous	3.6
Zinc	2.8

You might have heard that eggs are linked to heart disease. This is a myth—thirty years of scientific research has yet to link the two. In fact, a study completed in 2007 shows that, although eggs do not increase the chance of heart disease in healthy adults, they may be associated with a decrease in blood pressure (besides having tremendous nutritional value).

Chefs have long considered the mastery of egg cookery to be an excellent way to measure incoming chefs. Master French Chef Fernana Point (1897–1955) would test visiting chefs with a challenge to show him how they fried a simple egg, declaring that the easiest dishes were often the most difficult to prepare. When, inevitably, the new chef insulted the egg with the sizzling hot surface of a frying pan, Point would cry, "Stop, unhappy man, you are making a dog's bed of it!"

Because you will likely be eating many eggs in your Fight Fat with Fat Diet and to make sure you know how to cook eggs more kindly, I give you the following twelve recipes for the basic egg dishes.

Soft-cooked Eggs

For each person, place two large eggs in a small bowl of warm tap water to cover. Fill a small saucepan three-quarters full of water. Raise to a boil and then add a pinch of salt. Lower the eggs on a spoon into gently boiling water. Cook 4 minutes for a soft center and 6 minutes for medium. Lift eggs out with a spoon, run under cold tap water a moment, then transfer to an eggcup. Nip the end of the egg off with a knife and dive in.

Hard-cooked Eggs

For each person, place two large eggs in a small bowl of warm tap water to cover. Fill a small saucepan three-quarters full of water. Raise to a boil and then add a pinch of salt. Lower the eggs on a spoon into gently boiling water. Cook 10 minutes. You can also place eggs in the pan of water to begin. Once the eggs are cooked, plunge them into cold water. Once they have cooled, crack and shell them, and now you are ready for devilled eggs, egg salad, or endless garnishes and nutritional boosts to salads.

Poached Eggs

The beauty of poached eggs is that you can cook as many as 15 at a time if you are having a party or you can just cook yourself a couple. The key is to use the freshest possible eggs so they will hold their shape. In at least four inches of simmering water with a tablespoon of vinegar, gently slip the eggs into the water and watch until the white has set up and the yolk looks firm. Use a slotted spoon to lift them from the water. Hold a towel in your other hand, and let the excess water drip off, then slide the egg into a bowl.

Coddled Eggs

No, these eggs have not been hugged and kissed, but rather are cooked in cute little porcelain dishes available at any cooking-supply store. Brush the dish with butter, break the eggs in, screw on the metal top, and lower into barely boiling water. Cook 7 to 8 minutes; then lift out of the water. Use tongs; do not lift through the ring on the top. Place the porcelain coddlers on a plate and serve. What that gets coddled is the person who eats them. Makes you feel so special.

Oeufs en Cocotte

This is French for eggs baked in a dish. Simply use any small ramekin or baking dish, slather it with butter, break a couple eggs in, season with salt and pepper, add a splash of cream on top, and place it in a 325° oven for about 12 to 14 minutes. Transfer the dish to a plate and serve. I think of this kind of egg cookery as a lot of sizzle for the simple egg.

Microwaved Eggs

Do not try cooking eggs in the shells in the microwave unless you are interested in science experiments regarding the difficulty of removing cooked egg from the walls of the oven. They will explode. However, you can make quick and easy scrambled eggs. Place two eggs in a well-buttered 10-ounce custard cup. Season to taste with salt and pepper. Add 1 tablespoon cream and whisk with a fork. Cook uncovered from 1 to 2 minutes, whisking once in the middle, but just until liquid egg is no longer visible. Then remove from the oven and cover and let stand for a minute or so. Now that is a pretty quick meal. Three minutes tops.

Fried Eggs

Now this is all about the pan, a fresh egg, some butter, and the correct temperature. You have probably been served eggs that had a whiff of burnt hair and crispy icky edges. That was a result of a too-hot pan.

Frying eggs should be simple. Preheat a perfectly clean heavy skillet over medium heat. Then add butter and swirl to melt it. Break eggs into the pan, reduce heat to low, add a teaspoon of water, cover and wait a minute. Open up the lid. The eggs should be just about cooked, whites set, yolk looking shiny. Transfer to a plate, season with salt and pepper, and eat.

Scrambled Eggs

Choose an 8- to 10-inch heavy skillet. Preheat over medium heat. Meanwhile, whisk a couple of eggs with a teaspoon of water and salt and pepper. Add a knob of butter to the pan and swirl to melt it. Pour in the eggs, and reduce heat to low. Cook, stirring from time to time, until the eggs look a bit like runny cottage cheese.

Take care not to overcook or you will have a bad version of yellow rubber boots that smell something like burning hair. The eggs should clump up when you run the spatula under them, and once you see there is no more wet egg, quickly transfer them to your warmed breakfast plate.

Pickled Eggs

Hemingway considered the pickled eggs on the bar in one of his famous short stories. Nothing could be simpler to make.

   1 dozen eggs
   1 quart malt or cider vinegar (remember to avoid vinegar if
       you have a yeast problem)
   2 tablespoons freshly grated ginger
   1 tablespoon black peppercorns
   1 teaspoon allspice or pickling spice
   Hard cook the eggs. Shell them and place them in a half-
       gallon jar.

Combine the other ingredients in a saucepan with 1 cup water and raise to a rolling boil. Transfer to a large jar. Add the boiled and peeled eggs. Cover and refrigerate at least 24 hours or up to 1 month.

   When you need a quick pick-me-up, eat yourself a pickle.

Perfect Omelets

Get yourself a nice, new 8- to 12-inch omelet pan (a very clean nonstick pan will also suffice, but do not use Teflon). Which size pan you use depends upon your particular view of the omelet. If you are of the "you can't be too rich or too thin" school, choose the larger pan. If you prefer your omelet fluffy and a little thicker, choose the smaller. Purists will tell you the omelet should have NO browning but should simply be golden yellow. Personally, I like a little color on my omelet, not only for the look of it, but because the browning also complicates the flavor.

Next, prepare the filling. If you are grating cheese, use a microplane and grate it right onto the dinner plate you will ultimately use. Then, preheat the skillet over medium low heat.

Whisk 2 eggs with salt and pepper and a teaspoon of water. Melt a knob of butter in the skillet, swirling to cover every inch. Pour the eggs into the skillet. Let them set without touching for a minute, then begin lifting the skillet on one side and then the other so the runny part in the middle can move to the side.

Pick up an edge and see if it is beginning to color up. Add grated cheese to half of it, use your spatula to fold it over itself to turn it in half, and remove to the plate. Now what could be simpler? All of this is done in under 5 minutes.

Deviled Eggs

  6 large eggs
  ½ teaspoon white wine vinegar (remember to avoid vinegar
      if you have a yeast problem)
  1 tablespoon sour cream
  1 tablespoon mayonnaise
  1 tablespoon minced shallot
  2 teaspoons capers, finely minced
  Salt
  Pepper
  Dash of cayenne pepper
  1 tablespoon minced fresh chives or dill

To hard-cook eggs, bring a pan of water to simmer. Gently lay
eggs in the water, return to simmer, and cook for 8 minutes. Drain
and cool eggs in ice water just until cool enough to handle. (This
keeps yolks perfectly yellow, and the shell slips off easily when the
eggs are slightly warm.) Peel eggs and chill again in ice water until
cooled. Slice eggs in half lengthwise and remove yolks. Mash yolks
with vinegar, sour cream, mayonnaise, shallot, capers, salt and
pepper to taste, cayenne pepper, and chives or dill. Add a dollop
to each cooked egg white.

Egg Salad

  6 large eggs, hard cooked and peeled
  ½ cup mayonnaise
  ½ teaspoon curry powder
  1 teaspoon pickle relish
  1 teaspoon minced onion
  Salt to taste
  Pepper to taste

Chop eggs into a bowl. Mix with mayonnaise, curry, pickle relish, onion, and salt and pepper to taste. Place in a bowl and cover. Refrigerate up to a week.

Other Fight Fat with Fat Detox Full Fat Fast Recipes

Besides the dozen egg recipes, I offer only a few others for the detox phase. The simplest thing to do is go to a great butcher and fish monger, look in the case, and buy yourself grass-fed meats and wild-caught fish and shell fish. At home, cook them in a pan with butter and/or olive oil, seasoned with a simple sprinkling of sea salt and cracked black pepper. You will have sumptuous dinners in under ten minutes, no matter what you choose, and because you have chosen high-quality foods to begin with, it will be simple to stay on the plan and eat well.

Saucy Vodka Chicken

This spicy, smoky chicken is perfect, whether you are cooking for yourself for weeknight dinners or for an impromptu party. Start with three chickens, whole or broken up into parts. If you bought whole chickens, you will have leftover backs for stock. These brightly flavored chicken pieces are the Tupperware lunch item. And do not worry about that vodka. Since it has no carbs, it is perfectly all right to use.

Makes 12 to 16 servings

1 cup soy sauce
½ cup vodka
3 packets sugar substitute (or to taste)
½ cup extra-virgin olive oil, divided
6 large cloves garlic, smashed
4 tablespoons Asian sesame oil
3 tablespoons ground cumin
1 teaspoon dried hot red-pepper flakes (or to taste)
6 chicken wings (2 pounds total)
6 chicken breasts, cut in half with skin and bones (4 pounds total)
6 chicken thigh-drumsticks (3 pounds total)

Lime wedges for accompaniment
½ lime

Stir together soy sauce, vodka, sugar substitute, oil, garlic, sesame oil, cumin, and red-pepper flakes in a large glass measure. Divide chicken pieces among large sealable bags, then divide marinade among bags, and seal, pressing out excess air. Put bags in a large bowl (in case of leaks) and marinate the chicken, chilled, 2 hours to overnight.

Put oven racks in upper and lower thirds of oven and preheat oven to 450°F. Brush 2 large shallow baking pans with oil. Divide chicken between pans, skin side down. Pour marinade into a wide 4-quart saucepan. Roast chicken in oven 12 minutes. Turn chicken over, switch the pans, and return to oven until cooked through and lightly browned, 13 to 18 minutes more.

Transfer chicken to platter. While chicken roasts, gently boil marinade until reduced to about 1½ cups, 20 to 25 minutes. Drizzle chicken with some of the sauce and serve the remainder on the side with the lime wedges. Squeeze juice from lime half all over chicken before serving.

Leftover sauce keeps in an airtight container, chilled, up to 3 days. Cool completely, uncovered, then chill, covered. Bring to room temperature before using.

Per serving: CALORIES 460, FAT 34 g., PROTEIN 35.6 g., CARBS 7.2 g., FIBER 1.2 g.

Sautéed Flank Steak with Anchovy Sauce

Here is French cooking 101: a simple steak cooked and fanned out onto the plate in a mouthwatering presentation. If you prefer another cut, feel free to substitute. Anything from a skirt to a filet mignon works well.

Makes 4 servings

1 flank steak, about 16 ounces
Juice of 1 lime
Kosher salt to taste
Cracked black pepper to taste
Whiff cayenne pepper
2 tablespoons extra-virgin olive oil
1 2-ounce can anchovies in oil (reserve oil)
6 large cloves garlic, smashed
1 green onion and top, minced
½ cup water

Rub steak with 1 tablespoon lime juice and sprinkle with salt, pepper, and cayenne 10 minutes before cooking. Heat olive oil and oil from canned anchovies in large, heavy skillet over high heat. When hot, add steak and cook about 2 minutes on each side for medium rare, or to preferred doneness. When steak is cooked, transfer to a warmed plate to rest a few minutes.

Meanwhile, crush anchovy fillets with garlic. Add to green onion in the pan drippings and cook about 30 seconds. Add water and boil 30 seconds, wiping up bits from the bottom of the pan. Swirl butter into the pan to melt. Pour over steak, sprinkle with more lime juice, and cut into thin slices and serve on warmed plates.

Per serving: CALORIES 265, FAT 15.3 g., PROTEIN 28.5 g., CARBS 1.9 g., FIBER .02 g.

Bourbon Chicken Liver Pâté

If you would like to create your own luxury on a diet, make a pan of this pâté, refrigerate it, and eat a 2-ounce slice every three hours.
Makes 8 to 10 servings

1½ sticks (¾ cup) unsalted butter, divided
1 cup finely chopped onion
1 large garlic clove, minced
1 teaspoon minced fresh thyme or ¼ teaspoon dried
1 teaspoon minced fresh marjoram or ¼ teaspoon dried
1 teaspoon minced fresh sage or ¼ teaspoon dried
Sea salt to taste
Black pepper to taste
⅛ teaspoon ground allspice
1 pound chicken livers
2 tablespoons bourbon
Sprig of fresh thyme, marjoram, or sage for garnish
Special equipment: a 2½-cup crock or terrine or several
   small ramekins

Melt 1 stick butter in a large nonstick skillet over moderately low heat, and then cook onion and garlic, stirring, until softened, about 5 minutes. Add herbs, salt, pepper, allspice, and livers and cook, stirring until livers are cooked outside but still pink when cut open, about 8 minutes.

Stir in bourbon and remove from heat. Purée mixture in a food processor until smooth; then transfer pâté to crock and smooth the top.

Melt remaining ½ stick butter in a very small heavy saucepan over low heat; then remove pan from heat and let butter stand 3 minutes. If using herb garnish, put sprig on top of pâté. Skim froth from butter, then spoon enough clarified butter over pâté to cover its surface, leaving milky solids in bottom of pan.

Chill pâté until butter is firm, about 30 minutes; then cover with plastic wrap and chill at least 2 hours more.

Per serving: CALORIES 187, FAT 16 g., PROTEIN 8 g., CARBS 1.5 g., FIBER .4 g.

Apple-smoked Pork Loin

Pork loin is an easy meat to cook and keep on hand in the refrigerator for quick lunches during the week.

Makes 8 servings

3 cups apple-wood or orange-wood chips or 6 to 8 apple-wood
   or orange-wood chunks
2- to 2½-pound boneless pork top loin roast (single loin)
2 teaspoons dried oregano, crushed
4 cloves garlic, minced
½ teaspoon sea salt, or to taste
½ teaspoon freshly milled black pepper, or to taste

At least 1 hour before cooking, soak wood chips or chunks in enough water to cover. Meanwhile, trim fat from roast. Place roast in a shallow dish. In a small bowl, stir together dried oregano, garlic, salt, and pepper. Sprinkle evenly over all sides of roast; rub in with your fingers.

Drain wood chips. Prepare grill for indirect grilling. Test for medium-low heat above drip pan. Sprinkle half of the drained wood chips over the coals.

Place roast on grill rack directly over drip pan. Cover and grill for 1 to 1½ hours or until internal temperature registers 155°F on an instant-read thermometer. Add more coals and remaining wood chips as needed during grilling.

Remove roast from grill. Cover with foil; let stand for 15 minutes. The temperature of the meat will rise 5°F during standing. To serve, slice pork.

Per serving: CALORIES 190, FAT 9 g., PROTEIN 24 g., CARBS 5.3 g., FIBER .01 g.

Pork Medallions in Capers

Choose boneless pork medallions for ease of use, or make thin slices from a pork tenderloin. This is on the table in less than 10 minutes.

Makes 4 servings

1 pound pork medallions
Kosher salt to taste
Freshly milled black pepper to taste
2 tablespoons extra-virgin olive oil
¼ cup chicken broth
3 tablespoons capers, drained
2 tablespoons fresh lemon juice
Grated zest of ½ lemon

Pound pork between wax paper to ¼-inch thickness. Season with salt and pepper. Heat oil in a large skillet over medium-high heat, then cook pork, 2 minutes to the side, or until browned.

Add broth, capers, and lemon and cook 2–3 minutes, or until liquid has reduced by half. Serve hot.

Nutritional readout: CALORIES 168, FAT 7.4 g., PROTEIN 23.3 g., CARBS 1.3 g., FIBER .3 g.

Grilled Pesto Lamb Chops

Bright Mediterranean flavors bring hints of the Middle East to these luscious chops.

Makes 4 servings

1 cup fresh basil leaves
1 tablespoon grated Parmesan
2 teaspoons pine nuts
2 cloves garlic, smashed
2 tablespoons Greek yogurt
4 4-ounce lamb chops
Kosher salt
Freshly milled black pepper
1 tablespoon extra-virgin olive oil

Position knife blade in food processor bowl; add basil, Parmesan, pine nuts, and garlic. Process until smooth. Transfer mixture to a small bowl; stir in yogurt. Cover and chill 30 minutes.

Heat grill; then coat grill rack with vegetable cooking spray. Season chops with salt and pepper and then cook 5 minutes per side or until medium rare. Serve with a dollop of pesto on each chop. Garnish with fresh basil sprigs.

Per serving: CALORIES 214, FAT 9.8 g., PROTEIN 27.8 g., CARBS 2.1 g., FIBER 1.2 g.

Super-easy Baked Ham

Start with a fully cooked ham, coat it with mustard, and you will have a treat that is delicious, hot or cold.

Makes 12 servings

1 6- to 8-pound cooked ham, bone-in shank half
Ballpark yellow mustard to coat the outside

Preheat oven to 350°F and make sure the racks are all the way on the bottom so there is plenty of room for the ham.

Take ham out of wrapper and rinse it with cool water. Place ham in pan with large cut side down. Make cross hatch mark in the skin and place it skin side up in a roasting pan. Coat with mustard.

Cook until internal temperature reaches 140°F. Set it aside to rest before carving.

Per serving: CALORIES 535, FAT 39.7 g., PROTEIN 41.3 g., CARBS 4.3 g., FIBER 2.0 g.

Branzino with Walnut Purée

Recipe courtesy of California Walnut Board, Chef Ethan Stowell of Union in Seattle. This is a quick and satisfying supper.

Makes 4 servings

1 cup California walnut pieces, toasted a moment in a dry skillet
¼ cup extra-virgin olive oil, plus 2–3 tablespoons
2 tablespoons finely chopped fresh chives
2 whole branzino (or white sea bass), cut into fillets, 4 total
Kosher salt
Freshly ground black pepper

To make the walnut purée, combine the walnuts and ¼ cup of olive oil in a food processor and process for about 1 minute, or until smooth (add more olive oil if needed). Scrape the walnut purée into a bowl, stir in the chives, and season with salt and pepper to taste. Set aside.

Rub the fish with 2–3 tablespoons of olive oil, and season both sides with salt and pepper. Just before you cook the fish, place about 2 tablespoons of the walnut purée in the center of 4 dinner plates. Grill the fish 2–3 minutes on each side. Place a fish fillet on each plate, over the walnut purée.

Per serving: CALORIES 482, FAT 36.5 g., PROTEIN 35.8 g., CARBS 4.0 g., FIBER .6 g.

Seared Scallops with Gremolata

Choose large, meaty sea scallops for ease of preparation, and remember this gremolata, which is simply a Mediterranean mix of fresh herbs, works well with other protein choices as well: lamb, chicken, turkey. Make the recipe work for you.

Makes 4 servings

1½ pounds large sea scallops
Sea salt to taste
Freshly milled black pepper to taste
1 tablespoon extra-virgin olive oil, divided
1 shallot, minced
½ cup dry white wine
Juice and grated zest of 1 lemon
1 tablespoon minced Italian parsley
1 tablespoon minced chives
1 tablespoon minced basil

Season scallops with salt and pepper on a paper towel. Heat half the oil in a large skillet and then sear the scallops until brown on the edges, about 3–4 minutes. Move to a warm dish.

Add remaining oil and shallot and sauté 1 minute. Add wine, lemon juice and zest, parsley, chives, and basil. Heat 1 minute and then pour over scallops and serve.

Per serving: CALORIES 175, FAT 3.7 g., PROTEIN 28.8 g., CARBS 4.3 g., FIBER .3 g.

Seared Cod with Browned Butter and Almonds

Any cold-water, firm-fleshed fish will work with this recipe. You will be getting lots of omega-3 and omega-6 fatty acids, as well as fantastic flavor.

Makes 4 servings

4 6-ounce cod fillets
Kosher salt to taste
Freshly milled black pepper to taste
3 tablespoons butter
¼ cup sliced almonds
Juice and grated zest of ½ lemon

Season fish with salt and pepper. Heat a skillet to medium high, and then add butter. After it has melted, sauté the fish until golden on each side, adding almonds the last minute. Add lemon juice and zest and stir. Place the fish on a plate and pour the sauce over it.

Per serving: CALORIES 226, FAT 9.8 g., PROTEIN 31.7 g., CARBS 1.9 g., FIBER .8 g.

Lemon Yellow Tail with Tomato-dill Sauce

This popular Gulf of Mexico fish is a cousin to Amberjack and mild flavored and wonderful with sauces. As always, substitute whatever you find in the case that is really fresh.

Makes 4 servings

4 6-ounce yellow tail fillets
2 tablespoons yellow mustard
Kosher salt to taste
Freshly milled black pepper to taste
2 tablespoons extra-virgin olive oil
¼ cup minced green onions
1 plum tomato, minced
Juice and grated zest of 1 lemon
½ cup dry white wine
2 tablespoons butter

Rub mustard, salt, and pepper over fish on both sides. Heat oil in a large skillet and sauté fish until golden, about 5 minutes. Remove to a warm plate. Add green onions, tomato, and lemon juice and zest to the pan and cook about 1 minute. Add wine and cook down by half. Swirl in butter to make a sauce, and pour over fish and serve.

Per serving: CALORIES 235, FAT 8.2 g., PROTEIN 34.6 g., CARBS 4.2 g., FIBER 0.6 g.

Curry-orange Salmon

Citrus and curry make a splendid sweet, sour, hot, and sassy flavor note for the ubiquitous salmon. Remember to buy only wild-caught salmon, never farm raised.

Makes 4 servings

¼ cup chopped cilantro
3 tablespoons extra-virgin olive oil, divided
1 tablespoon curry powder
Juice and grated zest of 1 orange
Salt to taste
Freshly milled black pepper to taste
1½ pounds salmon sides
Orange wedges

Stir together cilantro, 1 tablespoon oil, curry, orange juice and zest, salt, and pepper. Paste it onto the fish. Heat remaining oil in a large skillet and sauté fish until golden, about 4 minutes. Serve with orange wedges.

Per serving: CALORIES 308, FAT 16.6 g., PROTEIN 36.3 g., CARBS 1.7 g., FIBER .3 g.

Grilled Salmon Provencal with Yogurt Sauce

Salmon steaks are great for this satisfying 10-minute dinner.
Makes 4 servings

½ cup Greek yogurt
2 garlic cloves, minced
Kosher salt to taste
Freshly milled black pepper to taste
4 6-ounce salmon steaks
2 tablespoons extra-virgin olive oil
2 cups cherry tomatoes, halved
3 tablespoons basil, cut chiffonade

Stir together yogurt, garlic, salt, and pepper. Set it aside. Season tuna with more salt and pepper. Heat a large skillet with oil and sauté tuna steaks until golden, about 3 minutes per side. Remove to a warm plate. Add tomatoes and basil to the pan and heat for 3 minutes or so until soft. Mound tuna and tomatoes on a plate and top with a dollop of the yogurt mixture.

Per serving: CALORIES 256, FAT 6.5 g., PROTEIN 43.1 g., CARBS 4.8 g., FIBER 1.1 g.

Bone Broth

Dr. Weston A. Price, the dentist who roamed the earth studying native cultures in the early part of the twentieth century, was the first one to record the ravages of the Western diet in his book, *Nutrition and Physical Degeneration*, first published in 1939 and in continual publication since. Dr. Price recorded cultures from the Amazon to the Arctic, noting the diets of native peoples before and after they had been introduced to the so-called Western diet. He concluded that much of the so-called modern diet was impacting the health of people around the world. "Life in all its fullness is mother nature obeyed," said Dr. Price. For a great resource and for sound nutritional advice, log onto www.westonaprice. org, including dates for the annual conference, which provides a wealth of information.

This basic broth recipe is found in traditional cultures from Eastern Europe to South America. We use this broth as the basis for soups, to start meals, and to build up our immune systems. Not only is it good for us; it also tastes good.

Buy chicken backs and beef neck bones and combine the two to make this healthy broth.

Makes about one gallon

2–4 pounds raw chicken or beef bones
2 tablespoons apple-cider vinegar
1 gallon water
1 onion, cut in chunks
1 head of garlic, broken into cloves and smashed

Simmer bones in water and vinegar at least 5 hours. The bones will soften, and the vinegar helps release minerals into the broth. When broth is cool, skim off fat, strain, and store broth in ziplock bags in the freezer.

Per cup: CALORIES 55, FAT 1.2 g., PROTEIN 5.1 g., CARB 0.5 g., FIBER 0.

Lemon Water

In the 1940s, a craze, called the Master Cleanse, swept outward from Hollywood. Basically, it was a fast that had people drink lemon water with a shot of cayenne for days on end to detoxify their bodies. Although, I do not recommend restricting yourself to lemon water alone, I do believe it is a healthy addition to the Fight Fat with Fat Diet Detox.

> 1 8-ounce glass ice water
> Juice of ½ lemon
> Whiff of cayenne
> Stevia to sweeten

Stir and enjoy. You could drink four of these a day, and you would not only lose weight but also build your immune system with the super charge of vitamin C you get.

Per serving: CALORIES 1.3, FAT 0, PROTEIN 0, CARBS .4 g., FIBER 0.

Full-fat Chocolate Ice Cream

No need to give up ice cream. The flavor with all-natural stevia is fantastic. You can substitute other flavorings for the cocoa: lemon zest and juice, orange, crushed coffee beans, a vanilla bean, or smashed berries of your choice.

Makes 1 quart

4 large organic egg yolks
4 cups heavy cream
¼ cup best quality unsweetened cocoa
Pinch salt
8–10 drops liquid stevia (or to taste)

Whip egg yolks and half the cream in a glass measure or bowl. Pour remaining cream, cocoa, and salt in a heavy-bottom saucepan and heat until cocoa is completely dissolved.

Pour custard and cocoa mixture together and whisk thoroughly. Cook until the custard coats the back of a spoon. Cover and refrigerate at least 4 hours. Pour the mixture into the ice cream canister and freeze in your ice cream maker.

Per serving: CALORIES 454, FAT 47.3 g., PROTEIN 4.3 g., CARBS 6.2 g., FIBER 8 g.

Classic Custard

Here is a foolproof dessert for you to make and refrigerate until you really need a sweet finish to dinner. It even works well as a snack. You can gild it further with a dollop of whipped cream if you wish.

Makes 6 servings

4 cups (1 quart) heavy cream
6 large eggs, separated
¼ teaspoon cream of tartar
¼ teaspoon salt
6 packets sugar substitute (or to taste)
2 teaspoons vanilla extract
1 teaspoon almond extract
Ground cinnamon on top
Blueberries, strawberries, or raspberries for garnish

Preheat the oven to 325°F. Spritz a 4-quart casserole or 6 individual ramekins with buttery cooking spray and set aside. Place a large pan with 1 inch of water in the middle of the lower rack of the oven to preheat.

Pour cream into a microwave-safe bowl and heat at 100-percent power for 4 minutes. Alternatively, heat on the stovetop to just under the boiling point.

Meanwhile, beat egg whites with cream of tartar and salt until soft peaks form.

In a large separate bowl, beat egg yolks with sweetener until well blended and then pour in hot cream and beat a moment. Season with vanilla and almond extracts. Fold beaten egg whites into this mixture.

Pour into prepared casserole or ramekins, top with a sprinkling of ground cinnamon, cover with buttered parchment paper, place in the water bath, and bake 45 to 50 minutes, or until a knife inserted in the middle comes out clean.

Serve custard warm or cold in a dessert dish with a side of fresh berries. Top with whipped cream if you wish.

Per serving: CALORIES 289, FAT 22 g., PROTEIN 10.2 g., CARBS 10.9 g., FIBER .4 g.

Cinnamon Soufflé

This is a perfect punctuation point to a divine dinner. Master souf-
flés and omelets, and you are on the way to becoming a fabulous
cook. This simple, lovely soufflé makes a satisfying end to a rich
country meal.

Choose the best cinnamon you can lay hands on for optimum
flavor. For the best flavor, use your microplane and grate the cinnamon yourself from whole cinnamon sticks.

Makes 8 ½-cup servings

12 ounces cream cheese
16 ounces sour cream or crème fraiche
8 drops stevia (or up to 6 packets) or to taste)
Pinch salt
½ teaspoon freshly grated cinnamon
8 large eggs, separated.

Separate the eggs. Heat oven to 300°F.

Thoroughly mix cream cheese, sour cream, stevia, salt, cinnamon, and egg yolks in a large bowl.

In a standing mixer, beat egg whites until stiff, then fold in the
egg yolk mixture. Divide among 8 ramekins or in a large soufflé
pan. Place ramekins on a baking sheet and then bake until golden
brown and puffed (about 18 minutes for individuals and 45 minutes for the large one).

Serve immediately. Once you are in the Marathon phase, add
a side of raspberries.

Per serving: CALORIES 333, FAT 28.5 g., PROTEIN 10.4 g.,
CARBS 5.8 g., FIBER 0.1 g.

French Chocolate Cake (Flourless)

Serve warm or cold with whipped cream. The cream may be sweetened with stevia and dusted with cocoa powder before serving. For the Marathon phase, add a few berries on the side.

Makes 12 servings

½ cup Dutch-process European pure unsweetened cocoa
6 ounces 70% cacao dark chocolate
1 cup unsalted butter
10 packets (or to taste) stevia
4 large eggs, separated

Preheat oven to 350°F. Line one 9-inch, removable-bottom cake tin with parchment paper and generously coat the paper with butter.

Break the chocolate into pieces and melt them with butter and cocoa over hot water stirring with a rubber spatula.

Beat the egg yolks with the sugar substitute until light. Fold in the melted butter and chocolate mixture.

Beat egg whites until stiff peaks form. Fold into chocolate mixture. Pour into the prepared pan.

Bake until a wooden pick inserted in center comes out clean, approximately 40 minutes.

Use a knife to separate the cake from the paper. Please observe that the cake is quite sticky!

Per serving: CALORIES 263, FAT 23.2 g., PROTEIN 3.9 g., CARBS 9.8 g., FIBER 2.2 g.

PART III

THE FIGHT FAT WITH FAT MARATHON

EASY STEPS TO DIETING SUCCESS

The Road to Good Health, Normal Weight, and Long and Vigorous Life

Join the Fight Fat with Fat Marathon, and you can expect to lose two to five pounds a week, you will not feel hungry, and you should not suffer cravings. If you do, I will tell you what to do about them too.

As I have said before, the human body is amazingly adaptable, and just as it adapted to an eating pattern that packed on the pounds and threatened your health, given a chance, your body can heal itself. All you have to do is cooperate a bit.

The Marathon will reintroduce complex carbohydrates in a step-wise fashion. After your week or two in the Full Fat Fast detox, your body is now ready for the long haul. Whether you need to lose twenty pounds or two hundred, this Marathon will get you there.

I promised you would not have to count calories or worry about fat ever again, but you do need to be aware of carbohydrates and reintroduce complex carbohydrates in an orderly way so that you do not undo the good work you have done in the detox period. Keep in mind that complex carbohydrates are whole vegetables, fruits, and grains. Simple carbohydrates, such as sugars, flours, and processed foods, are not on your food list. And actually, they should never be, except for very special occasions.

OK. You can have a piece of cake on your birthday.

Be patient with yourself. This change takes time. Some people are more addicted than others to chips, cookies, soda, and all of the zillion and one bad-for-you foods. But the more you nourish your body with whole, organic foods, the less your body will be screaming for the bad stuff.

Remember, this is a tri-part system:

Diet
Exercise
Attitude

The more you experience success on the Fight Fat with Fat Diet, the more success you will continue to have. You have already succeeded at the detox phase. I hope you have ramped up your exercise to the point that you are walking every day, and I am sure your attitude is improving because you are making positive changes in your body. Aim for ten thousand steps a day. Buy a pedometer. This is not as hard as it sounds.

You will have plenty of energy, you will feel good, you will look good, and you will achieve your dietary goals. Add a simple weight-lifting regimen to your week. Two to three times a week, lift five-pound weights in a program to increase your upper-body strength. Go to a gym, hire a personal trainer, or buy an appropriate video to guide you. If you are a beginner, start here: http://www.ehow.com/how_5199034_start-weight-training-women.html.

The Fight Fat with Fat Marathon

The Fight Fat with Fat Marathon is a progression into a broad and varied diet of organic whole foods for health, weight loss, and long life. It has simple, easy-to-follow steps.

- Eat five meals a day. Pay attention to everything you eat. Control the portions.

- Drink plenty of water, at least sixty-four ounces, including tea and coffee.

- Exercise at least fifteen minutes every day.

- Sleep eight hours every night.

- Reduce stress in your life.

Eat Five Meals a Day

At first, you may notice that paying attention to everything you eat seems like a chore, but soon it will become second nature. Make a point of sitting down to eat, away from your desk, away from the telephone, away from the television. Be mindful of the food you put in your mouth.

This diet is made up of the finest, purest foods there are. It is a luxury to eat this way. You deserve the very best, and this diet gives that to you. Make a conscious choice not to eat junk food. Eliminate white flour and sugar from your diet in all combinations.

Portion control is perhaps the biggest challenge for those of us who have been living on the so-called Western diet in which the super-sized portions have created a nation of overfed, under-nourished people. If you learn to manage your portions, you will not have to count calories. Buy yourself a food scale and weigh meats and cheeses to get accustomed to serving sizes. This will help you when you go out to eat where most portions are at least twice and sometimes three times the amount of food needed for nourishment.

3 ounces of meat is about the size of a deck of cards
1 ounce of cheese is about the size of a domino

Making your metabolism work better and regulating your glucose depends on regular, small servings of high-protein, high-fat meals. This will stop your cravings in their tracks. You will not get those desperate urges for junk food from the machine or the deli down on the corner. Every day:

- Eat five meals.

- For breakfast, eat two eggs.

- Twice a day, have four to five ounces of fish or meat.

- Morning and evening, enjoy small snacks of nutrient-dense cheese, nuts, olives, jerky, ham, or turkey.

Becoming mindful of one's body is often a new thing for people who have been overweight for years. They have never experienced their body as being "empty" of food. Instead, they only thought they were feeling hunger when they were really confusing it with hypoglycemia—a state where the blood sugars have dropped precipitously, warning that the body is about to go into shock.

A body that is well nourished and receiving sufficient protein on a regular basis throughout the day will regulate itself. On the Fight Fat with Fat Diet, you will burn fat. You will never feel hungry. You can trust your body, which, given a chance, can regulate itself. You will soon cast long, loving looks at yourself in the mirror because you will look GREAT.

Drink Plenty of Water

Start your day with a hot cup of tea or coffee. This stimulates the digestive system and will help you to feel full faster. If you have trouble drinking the amount of water you need, buy yourself a sixty-four-ounce sports bottle and fill it up. By the end of the day, make sure you have drunk every drop. Because drinking water before a meal helps you to feel fuller, when you sit down at a restaurant, ask for water and drink the whole glass before the food arrives. At home, add a squeeze of lemon juice and a shot of cayenne for a full detox effect.

Exercise at Least Fifteen Minutes a Day

Now that many of us are planted in front of a computer for eight or more hours a day, the notion of exercise may seem impossible. But, if you stop and think of your normal day's activities, you may see how you can tuck in some exercise without too much effort. If you sit at a computer terminal, get up and walk for five minutes every hour. Try running up and down a flight of stairs—just for the fun of it.

Aim to set aside at least fifteen minutes every day for vigorous walking. Add exercise time and increase the rigor as you are able. You do not have to go crazy here with an exercise program. Walk your dogs. Walk on your lunch hour. Park in the spot FARTHEST from the mall. If you have an exercise bike in the basement, jump on it for fifteen minutes. Whatever you do, try to get your heart rate up and pounding. Try to walk ten thousand steps during your day. (Use a pedometer. I like the Omron.)

You may already be getting strength training in your daily life. Do you have a toddler you are carrying around? Are you hauling groceries in the house on a daily basis? Pushing a heavy vacuum cleaner? Gardening? All of these exercises build strength. But for a more focused exercise plan, give yourself fifteen minutes a day. OK, go ahead; multitask. Watch the news on TV while you are making yourself stronger. Use a couple of three-pound weights and do some lifts and pull ups. Use an exercise rope and do some bicep curls or front raises. Start out doing ten and work up to twenty-five reps.

Lie on the floor and do some old-fashioned sit ups. Start with ten and work up to twenty. Just feel the burn and keep at it. You will make yourself stronger.

The quickest way to get started is to hire a personal trainer for a few sessions. Work with your trainer to establish a routine that works for you.

Sleep Eight Hours Every Night

Get a full eight hours of rest every night. No matter what. Feeling insomniac? Try drinking two tablespoons of cream.

Reduce Stress in Your Life

The exercise you do will contribute to reducing stress, as well as strengthen your muscles. In addition and also to combat fatigue, try participating in activities you find fun, such as sports or hiking. Spending time in nature especially soothes the spirit. Join a class to learn meditation. Try yoga that emphasizes internal work, rather than physical exercise. Signing up for a class helps keep you committed to the program.

Check Your Progress

Assess yourself. Have you lost five to fifteen pounds? Has your waist size dropped two to four inches? Check your BMI (http://www.cdc.gov/healthyweight/assessing/bmi/adult_bmi/english). Make sure it is on the downward run.

If you are a woman, is your waist measurement over thirty-five inches, or if a man, over forty inches? If so, you are still in the obese category and should stick with the Full Fat Fast, the Fight Fat with Fat Detox plan, another week or so or until you are out of the danger zone. We have had patients who stayed on the detox phase for months. No harm done. Eating out for lunch after a two-egg breakfast is easy. Order a chop, a steak, a fish steak or fillet, or some shrimp. See? Not so hard.

Case Study

When Paul came to see me, he was 120 pounds overweight. His cardiologist had told him he was headed for myocardial infarction, a.k.a. a heart attack. He began the Full Fat Fast program and ultimately stayed on it for a little over one month. In thirty-five days, Paul lost forty pounds and happily moved to the Marathon phase to continue his weight-loss program.

PHASES OF THE MARATHON

When you have graduated from detox, here is how to start your own Marathon to keep yourself on the Fight Fat with Fat Diet. Following this section, once again, I give you guidelines for foods to eat and foods to avoid. Similar to the list for the Fight Fat with Fat Detox Full Fat Fast, the list of foods to adore in the Marathon stage now has more items for you to enjoy.

Phase 1

Here is what you will do now.

- Keep carbs to a total of 20 grams per day. Start with 3 cups of salad greens, or 2 cups of salad plus 1 cup cooked vegetables (from the approved list) for the first week.

- Enjoy full-fat, raw-milk aged cheese, up to 4 ounces a day, a handful of olives, and half an avocado every day.

- Dress your salads with extra-virgin olive oil and vinegar or lemon juice.

- Eat as much meats, fish, or fowl as you wish, including that yummy skin and fat.

- Continue to drink 64 ounces of fluids without *any* sugar daily.

- Keep up the 15 minutes (at least) of walking every day.

- Be aware of when you are full. Be mindful. Pay attention. Eat only until you are satisfied, not until you are stuffed.

Phase 2

After a week or so:

- Add back more vegetables and fruits. By now, you should be eating nine servings of vegetables and fruits a day. As long as your weight continues to drop, you can stay at this level of consumption.

- Once you come with ten pounds of your goal weight, add back a few complex carbohydrates—a cup of oatmeal for breakfast or a piece of multigrain bread for lunch.

- Include these flavorful, nutrient-dense additives for snacks as needed: 10 olives, half a Hass avocado. 2–3 tablespoons lemon or lime juice, pork skins, string cheese, beef jerky.

- Always monitor your weight, and should you hit a plateau that holds for several weeks, simply give yourself a week of the Full Fat Fast again, and you will be back on track.

If you wish, check the nutrient data from the U.S. government, www.nal.usda.gov/fnic/foodcomp/search/. Also, Ask.com has a good, free online carb counter. Or buy yourself a carb counter book. We recommend *Dr. Atkins' New Carbohydrate Gram Counter* (paperback).

Try squeezing lemon into ice water with a bit of artificial sweetener and a whiff of cayenne for your own kicked-up beverage. Avoid diet sodas. Some studies have shown that they trick the body into behaving as if real sugar has been consumed. Do not risk it.

Phase 3

Once your marathon is well under way:

- You may add more salad, other vegetables, fresh cheeses, seeds, nuts, berries and other fruits, legumes, some starchy vegetables, and whole grains.
- Add breakfast meats to your morning eggs—nitrate-free bacon and sausages are fine.
- Be mindful of your weight, and if you hit a plateau, back up to the stage of the Marathon or detox phase where you succeeded before by cutting out any of the foods listed above, and your weight loss should begin again.
- Remember to keep moving. Try to get in ten thousand steps a day.
- Keep a positive attitude and you will succeed.

Portion Sizes for Your Fight Fat with Fat Marathon

Buy your produce from a farmer's market for best flavor and nutrition. Shop for whole, unprocessed foods at all times and organic if possible. Stay away from processed foods and most foods labeled "diet," which are often loaded with chemicals and unhealthy filler.

Read labels ardently. If any prepared food product has more than ten carb grams, just put it back, no matter how the product is billed. If the product has fewer than ten grams, you may have it, but the NET result should always be ten carb grams OR LESS per day.

Meat and Beans

Aim for at least 3-4 servings each day. Choose fresh, unprocessed meats and nitrate-free bacon and sausages whenever possible. No restriction on portions except for beans.

Item	One Serving Equals	Visual Equivalent
Meat, tofu	2–3 ounces	Billiard ball
Beans	⅓ cup cooked beans	Billiard ball
Nuts, seeds	¼ cup	One handful

Fruits and Vegetables

Aim for 5–9 total servings each day. Choose fresh fruits and vegetables whenever possible.

Item	One Serving Equals	Visual Equivalent
Raw fruit	½ cup raw or canned fruit; ¼ cup frozen fruit; ½ apple, 8 spears of asparagus, ½ Hass avocado, ¼ cup melon, 1 kiwi, 1 tangerine, 1 medium tomato	Billiard ball
Dried fruit	¼ cup	An egg

Item	One Serving Equals	Visual Equivalent
Raw vegetables	1 cup	Baseball
Cooked vegetables	½ cup cooked vegetable, ⅓ cup cooked corn, on or off the cob	Billiard ball

Dairy

Aim for 2–3 servings of calcium-rich foods each day. Choose light or heavy cream and, sour cream. Avoid low-fat or fat-free milk and cheeses. Pick full-fat, raw-milk cheeses

Item	One Serving Equals	Visual Equivalent
Cheese	1 ounce full fat or 1 thin slice	A pair of dice
Milk	½ cup	

Fats and Oils

Eat natural fats and cold-pressed oils as needed. Choose heart-healthy fats whenever possible. No solid margarine or vegetable oils, which are known as trans-fats. Expeller nut oils, extra-virgin olive oil, coconut oil, and sesame oil are all great.

Item	One Serving Equals
Fats and oils	1–2 tablespoons

Whole Grains

Once you have reached the last leg of the Marathon, where you are running full out and are within ten pounds of your goal weight, add back this category. Aim for 2–3 servings each day. Remember to eat all of the protein and fat you want, but STOP eating when you feel full. Do not gorge yourself.

Item	One Serving Equals
Bread	1 ounce whole wheat and mixed grains; 1 small slice, ½ bagel, ½ bun
Cooked Grains	½ cup cooked

Beverages

You need at least sixty-four ounces of liquid a day. That is eight eight-ounce glasses. Pure water is your best source, but any beverage with no added sugars will qualify—tea, coffee, broth, seltzers, etc. You can add stevia for sweetening to any, lemon and a touch of cayenne to water to give it a bit of pizzazz.

As your weight normalizes, add back the complex carbohydrates. In the beginning, restrict yourself to fewer than 20 grams of carbohydrate grams a DAY. Then you can increase that up to nine servings, or 4½ cups, a day. Start with leafy green vegetables and berries, then gradually add in fruits, and finally add whole grains.

Think of it this way.

- Phase 1: Begin by aiming for 20 carbohydrate grams limit per day. You will lose 2-5 pounds per week.

- Phase 2: Once you come within 15 pounds of goal weight, you can ramp it up to 40 carbohydrate grams per day, and you can expect to lose 1 to 2 pounds per week.

- Phase 3: Once you are within 5 pounds of goal weight, push it up to 60 carbohydrate grams and include whole wheat bread (1 slice), brown rice (½ cup), or whole-wheat pasta (½ cup). Now is when you can enjoy that occasional piece of cake or chocolate chip cookie. You will probably not lose much weight at 60 grams of carbohydrate, but now you know what you should be doing for the rest of your life.

You can find great recipes in magazines and books. Just read the nutritional readout and watch out for hidden carbs. They are your enemy now and forever more.

When you follow the Fight Fat with Fat Marathon, your appetite will change. You will look at a plate of food with a different eye. You will not even consider that pile of pasta. You will just enjoy a half cup. Buckets of rice? I do not think so. Once you are near your goal weight, you will be satisfied with half a cup. This will be easy. I promise. You are on your Fight Fat with Fat for life.

The great thing about the Marathon is that you have changed your habits; you now understand what it takes to live a long and healthy life. You design your own eating plan and, so, design your life.

This time you can really do it!

FOODS TO ADORE

Be a label reader. Many so-called diet foods are loaded with carbohydrates. Do not be fooled. Read the fine print. If a food product has more than ten grams of carbohydrates, put it back.

Remember always to select foods that are sustainable, organic if possible, and whole and unprocessed.

Fats	Extra-virgin olive oil, butter, unrefined flaxseed oil, coconut oil, fresh lard, foie gras, nuts (walnuts, pecans, Brazil nuts, and hazelnuts).
Proteins	Organic or grass-fed beef, pork, veal, lamb, game, chicken, turkey, duck and other fowl (where possible). Chicken or veal liver, nitrate-free bacon and sausage, all seafood from cold, deep water (including codfish, halibut, and salmon), shellfish, and eggs.
Dairy	Organic and from pasture-fed cows: butter, raw-milk cheeses, full-fat or whipping cream, Greek yogurt, buttermilk, sour cream.

Vegetables	Organic salad vegetables: arugula, cabbage, celery, chicory, chives, cucumber, daikon, endive, escarole, fennel, jicama, lettuces, mache, mushrooms, parsley, peppers, radicchio, radishes, scallions, sorrel, spinach, sprouts of all kinds, tomato, watercress. Cooked organic vegetables: artichokes (whole or hearts), asparagus, bamboo shoots, bean sprouts, beet greens, bok choy, broccoli, broccoli rabe, Brussels sprouts, cabbage, cauliflower, celery root, chard, collard greens, dandelion greens, eggplant, hearts of palm, kale, kohlrabi, leeks, okra, onion, pumpkin, rhubarb, sauerkraut, snow peas, spaghetti squash, string or wax beans, summer squash, tomato, turnip, water chestnuts, zucchini. Organic berries in the beginning; then later add organic stone fruits (pears, peaches, plums, nectarines).
Beverages	Water (bottled waters of all kinds without added sugars), lemon water, coffee, herb tea, broth, club soda and seltzers without added sugars. Use stevia or Splenda to sweeten.
Condiments	Kosher or sea salt, black and red pepper, best quality balsamic vinegar, apple cider vinegar, rice wine vinegar, mayonnaise, mustards, soy sauce, fish sauce. Also crumbled bacon, caponata, grated hard cheeses, minced hard-cooked eggs, herbs, horseradish, sautéed mushrooms, pesto, pickles without sugar, prepared salad dressings with no carbs, shiritake or Miracle Noodles, spices, tamari, Tabasco, tapenade, Worcestershire sauce.

FOODS TO ABHOR

Fats	Highly processed vegetable oils (such as canola or soybean), margarine, vegetable shortening, all trans-fats (often found in processed foods and snacks).
Proteins	Processed meats.
Dairy	Processed cheeses, reduced or non-fat dairy products.
Carbohydrates	Any highly processed carbohydrate, white flour or anything made from white flour (including bread, cookies, crackers, pastas, and dry cereals), high fructose corn syrup, refined sugar, irradiated or genetically modified grains, chocolate mixed with sugar in any form.
Beverages	Soda, fruit juices, beer, wine, rice milk.
Condiments	Catsup, commercial baking powder, MSG, artificial flavors, artificial additives, and artificial colors.

MARATHON RECIPES AND MENU SUGGESTIONS

Thai Beef Lettuce Wraps

The brightly flavored recipes of Thailand have been widely adored in this country. No wonder. Yum.

.1 pound ground sirloin
1 tablespoon dark sesame oil, divided
2 tablespoons minced fresh ginger
¼ cup soy sauce
1 tablespoon rice vinegar
½ teaspoon dark sesame oil
½ teaspoon red pepper flakes
½ cup minced green onions
¼ cup chopped fresh cilantro
3 tablespoons chopped fresh mint
8 iceberg lettuce leaves
1 Kirby cucumber, cut into fine slices

Heat a large skillet, film it with sesame oil, and then add beef and ginger. Sauté until beef is cooked through, about 5 minutes. Stir in soy sauce, rice vinegar, remaining sesame oil, and red pepper. Cook about a minute. Remove skillet from the heat, and add onions, cilantro, and mint. Divide among lettuce leaves and serve with sliced cucumbers.

Nutritional readout: 158 CALORIES, FAT 5.5 g., PROTEIN 23.7 g., CARBS 5 g., FIBER 1.3 g.

Shrimp and Mango, Butter-lettuce Wraps with Peanut-Sauce

Wrap lettuce around almost anything you used to use as a sandwich filling, and it will taste good and be good for you.

Makes 16 servings

1½ pounds chopped cooked shrimp
2 cups diced mango
Juice and grated zest from 3 limes
2 tablespoons finely chopped fresh mint
$^1/_3$ cup flaked, unsweetened coconut
16 butter lettuce leaves
½ cup bottled peanut sauce
2 tablespoons chopped roasted almonds
In a bowl, combine shrimp, mango, lime zest, half the lime juice, and mint.

Cook coconut in a small skillet just until fragrant, and then add to the shrimp mixture. Toss and divide among lettuce leaves.

Stir remaining lime juice into peanut sauce and drizzle over shrimp. Fold leaves into diaper-fold and serve.

Nutritional readout: CALORIES 84, FAT 3 g., PROTEIN 7.1 g., CARBS 7.1 g., FIBER .8 g.

Chipotle Scallop Lettuce Wraps

Almost anything for a sandwich tastes great in a lettuce wrap. This goes for those wraps sold everywhere in diaper-folded flour tortillas (ugh). The flavor of these yummy shrimps in crisp butter lettuce is superior on all fronts. Enjoy.

Makes 4 servings

1 tablespoon cumin seeds
1 teaspoon chili powder
Sea salt to taste
Freshly milled black pepper to taste
1½ cups large scallops
2 tablespoons extra-virgin olive oil
2 cloves garlic, smashed
½ cup minced red onion
4 large butter lettuce leaves
½ cup chopped cilantro
Juice and grated zest from 1 lime
4 teaspoons sour cream
4 tablespoons chipotle salsa

Combine cumin, chili powder, salt, and pepper. Toss scallops in this mixture. Heat oil in a large skillet. Add garlic and onion and cook a moment; then add scallops and cook until opaque and golden, about 3 minutes.

Divide among lettuce leaves and then top each with cilantro, lime juice and zest, sour cream, and salsa. Fold and enjoy.

Nutritional readout: CALORIES 272, FAT 11.2 g., PROTEIN 35.4 g., CARBS 5.5 g., FIBER .09 g.

Pan-grilled Fish with Chermoula

Moroccans use this brightly flavored sauce with meat, fish, and shrimp. Take your pick. The results are the same. Fantastic!
Makes 4 servings

2 garlic cloves, smashed
½ teaspoon kosher salt
¼ cup extra-virgin olive oil
Juice and grated zest of 1 lemon
2 tablespoons parsley
2 tablespoons cilantro
1 teaspoon smoked paprika
½ teaspoon ground cumin
½ teaspoon coriander
½ teaspoon red pepper
1½ pounds fish fillet or large peeled shrimp, chicken, or lamb
Olive oil for cooking

Combine garlic and salt with a fork to make a paste. Add oil, lemon, parsley, cilantro, paprika, cumin, coriander, and red pepper. Smear this paste on surfaces of the fish or meat. Cook on an olive-oil-coated pan or grill.

Nutritional readout: CALORIES 282, FAT 13.6 g., PROTEIN 23.9 g., CARBS 4.4 g., FIBER .5 g.

Gingered Tilapia with Baby Spinach

On the table in 10 minutes and only 3 grams of carbohydrates. Woo hoo!

Makes 4 servings

4 tilapia (or other mild fish) fillets, 6 ounces each
2½ tablespoons freshly grated ginger root
Kosher salt to taste
Black pepper to taste
About 2 tablespoons extra-virgin olive oil
1 small onion, minced
6 cups (2 packages) baby spinach
¼ cup chicken broth
¼ cup dry white wine
4 lemon wedges for garnish

Rub fish fillets with 2 tablespoons ginger, salt, and pepper. Heat 1½ tablespoons oil in a large skillet over medium-high heat. Cook fish 2–3 minutes on each side, or until opaque. Remove from the pan and keep warm.

Film the pan with oil and cook onions and remaining ginger for 1 minute. Increase heat to high. Add spinach and season with additional salt and pepper, chicken broth, and wine. Cook 3 minutes or until wilted.

Serve fish on a bed of spinach and garnish with a lemon wedge.

Nutritional readout: CALORIES 233, FAT 8 g., PROTEIN 35 g., CARBS 3 g., FIBER 1 g.

Sole à la Bonne Femme

Got to hand it to the French. They eat well, and all understand it is the reason French women always seem to be thin. Although the recipe calls for flounder fillet, substitute the freshest fish in your fish monger's case. Pick what you love.

Makes 4 servings in less than 20 minutes

4 flounder (or other) fish fillets, about 1 pound
Kosher salt
Cracked black pepper
1 cup dry white wine
3 tablespoons butter
3 tablespoons shallots or green onions, minced, divided
½ pound sliced chanterelle (or button) mushrooms
¼ cup heavy cream
1 large egg yolk

Heat oven to 350°F. Butter a baking dish generously. Salt and pepper the fish and lay it in the dish. Pour wine over and bake, covered, about 10 minutes, or just until cooked through.

Pour the pan juices into a saucepan with butter, 2 tablespoons shallots, and mushrooms. Heat to boiling.

Meanwhile whisk cream and egg yolk together and then add to the sauce. To serve, pool sauce in a dinner sauce and add fish fillets. Garnish with remaining minced shallots and serve.

Nutritional Readout: CALORIES 349, FAT 22 g., PROTEIN 23 g., CARBS 3.3 g., FIBER .02 g.

Sautéed Shrimp on Red Cabbage with Parsley Sauce

Don't you just love one-dish dinners?

Makes 4 servings
6 tablespoons extra-virgin olive oil, divided
1 medium red cabbage, shredded (about 2 pounds)
Salt to taste
½ cup dry red wine
6 tablespoons unsalted butter
1 tablespoon minced onion
1 garlic clove, minced
4 tablespoons flat-leaf parsley, finely chopped
1½ pounds large peeled shrimp
Freshly milled black pepper to taste

Heat 2 tablespoons oil in a large skillet and add cabbage and a pinch of salt. Cook until cabbage begins to melt. Then add wine and cook and reduce 2–3 minutes more. Reduce heat to low; cover and cook until cabbage is tender, about 30 minutes. Adjust seasonings with salt. Transfer to a serving plate and cover.

Meanwhile, melt butter in a saucepan, add onion and garlic, and cook until soft, about 3 minutes. Remove from the heat and stir in parsley. Season with salt and 2 tablespoons oil and set it aside.

Heat 2 tablespoons oil in the skillet over medium heat. Cook shrimp just until it looks opaque, about 3 minutes. Season with salt and pepper.

To serve, mound cabbage on a plate and arrange shrimp around it, drizzling with parsley sauce.

Nutritional readout: CALORIES 304, FAT 1.22 g., PROTEIN 19.6 g., CARBS 9.6 g., FIBER 2.47 g.

Grilled Chili Shrimp with Avocado-orange Salsa

On the table in under 15 minutes, this flavorful Southwestern lunch is easy to make and really delicious.

Makes 4 servings

½ teaspoon ground cumin
1 teaspoon chili powder
Kosher salt to taste
Fresh ground black pepper to taste
1½ pounds large, peeled shrimp
1 large ripe Hass avocado, peeled, deseeded, and chopped
½ cup minced cilantro
2 cloves garlic, smashed
2 tablespoons minced green onion
2 tablespoons minced tomato
Juice and grated zest of one orange
2 tablespoons extra-virgin olive oil

Mix cumin, chili powder, salt, and pepper in a medium bowl. Dredge shrimp in the mixture.

Toss salsa ingredients together: avocado, cilantro, garlic, green onion, tomato, and juice and zest of the orange.

Heat oil in a large skillet and sauté shrimp until opaque and golden, about 3 minutes. To serve, mound salsa on a plate and top with shrimp.

Nutritional readout: CALORIES 242, FAT 12.6 g., PROTEIN 28.2 g., CARBS 5.4 g., FIBER 2.7 g.

Warm Salmon Salad with Caper Dressing

Quick as a wink and only 5 grams of carbohydrates.
Makes 4 servings

1 head butter lettuce
1 1-pound salmon fillet (about 1¼-inches thick)
½ teaspoon freshly ground black pepper
2 thick slices yellow onion
½ teaspoon dried or fresh dill weed
1 rib celery with leaves, minced
2 tablespoons mayonnaise
About 3 tablespoons lemon juice, divided
zest from ½ lemon
2 tablespoons water
1 tablespoon capers, drained

Line the bottom of the steamer rack with one lettuce leaf; then place the salmon, skin side down, on the lettuce. Season with pepper. Arrange onions around the fish. Sprinkle with dill. Cover and steam over boiling water 10–18 minutes, or until the fish is cooked through and opaque.* Do not overcook the fish. Once it loses its translucent look in the center, remove it to a plate.

While the fish and vegetables are cooking, use a fork to whisk together mayonnaise, 2 tablespoons lemon juice, lemon zest, water, and capers for the dressing.

Remove and discard the skin and bones from the cooked fish and break the fish into bite-sized chunks. Toss with the dressing.

To serve, arrange lettuce leaves on dinner plates, and divide the salad equally among 4 servings. Garnish each serving with a twist of lemon.

*In a hurry? Steam the fish on lettuce leaf in the microwave. Done in 3–4 minutes. Easy peezy.

Nutritional readout: CALORIES 303, FAT 20.8 g., PROTEIN 24.1 g., CARBS 5 g., FIBER 1.3 g.

Artichokes, Capers, Olives, Lemon Zest, and Salmon on Spaghetti Squash

In Italy, a no-cook pasta sauce is known as salsa cruda and makes a wonderful one-dish dinner. In this version, the combination of artichokes, olives, capers, and lemon zest is not only beautiful but also bold in flavor.

Makes 4 servings

1 spaghetti squash
1 6-ounce jar artichoke hearts, drained
¼ cup drained and rinsed capers
½ cup pitted and chopped Kalamata olives
Juice and zest of 1 lemon
1 16-ounce can salmon, drained
¼ cup extra-virgin olive oil
Freshly ground black pepper to taste
½ cup chopped fresh flat-leaf parsley leaves for garnish

Prick squash with a fork, then transfer to the microwave, and cook for 10–12 minutes.

Meanwhile, combine ingredients for salsa cruda in a medium bowl: artichoke hearts, capers, olive, lemon juice and zest, salmon, oil, and pepper.

Allow squash to cool a few minutes and then cut in half. Remove seeds. Using a fork, strip out spaghetti squash strings into a large serving bowl. Toss with salsa cruda. Garnish with chopped parsley leaves.

Nutritional readout: CALORIES 403, FAT 26.6 g., PROTEIN 22.1 g., CARBS 14.9 g., FIBER 3.2 g.

Dijon Egg and Salmon Salad

This flavor hit has everything in each bite: sweet, hot, bitter, salty, and crunchy. Served icy cold, it makes a terrific lunch.
Makes 2 servings

2 large eggs, hard cooked, peeled, and finely chopped
1 cup canned salmon, drained
¼ cup strawberries, chopped
2 tablespoons minced red onion
Grated zest of 1 lemon (about 1 teaspoon)
¼ cup toasted, slivered almonds
3 tablespoons mayonnaise
2 tablespoons Dijon mustard
Freshly milled black pepper to taste
6 leaves red-tipped lettuce
1 cup radish sprouts
Radishes for garnish

Stir together the chopped eggs, salmon, strawberries, onion, lemon zest, almonds, mayonnaise, and mustard. Season to taste with pepper. Cover and refrigerate until serving time.

To serve, spread egg-salmon salad onto a piece of ruffled red lettuce and sprouts. Serve garnished with radishes, as many as you want.

Nutritional readout: CALORIES 403, FAT 27 g., PROTEIN 33 g., CARBS 10 g., FIBER 4 g.

Coq au Vin

The classic French dish made famous by Julia Child in the sixties is still fabulous for those on the Fight Fat with Fat.

Makes 8 servings

½ pound bacon slices, coarsely chopped
20 pearl onions, peeled, or 1 large yellow onion, sliced
1 4-pound chicken, cut into serving pieces, or 3 pounds chicken parts, excess fat trimmed, skin on
6 garlic cloves, peeled
Salt to taste
Pepper to taste
2 cups chicken stock
2 cups red wine (Pinot Noir, Burgundy, or Zinfandel)
2 bay leaves
Several fresh thyme sprigs
Several fresh parsley sprigs, plus chopped fresh parsley for garnish
½ pound button mushrooms, trimmed and roughly chopped
2 tablespoons butter

Brown bacon on medium-high heat in a Dutch oven big enough to hold the chicken, until golden. Remove the cooked bacon; add onions and chicken, skin side down. Brown the chicken well, on all sides. Halfway through the browning, add the garlic and sprinkle the chicken with salt and pepper.

Spoon off any excess fat. Add the chicken stock, wine, and herbs. Add back the bacon. Lower heat to a simmer. Cover and cook for 20 minutes, or until chicken is tender and cooked through. Remove chicken and onions to a separate platter. Remove the bay leaves, herb sprigs, garlic, and discard. Add mushrooms to the remaining liquid and turn the heat to high. Boil quickly and reduce the liquid by three-fourths until it becomes thick and saucy. Lower the heat and stir in the butter. Return the chicken and onions to the pan to reheat and coat with sauce. Adjust seasoning. Garnish with parsley and serve.

Nutritional readouts: CALORIES 388, FAT 5.9 g., PROTEIN 23.8 g., CARBS 14.5 g., FIBER 2.1 g.

Chicken Breast in a Kalamata-caper Sauce

Boring chicken breasts need a lot of help. A shot of capers in a tomato pool is a good beginning. Plus it is on the table in less than 15 minutes. Yeah.

Makes 4 servings

4 boneless, skinless chicken breasts (4 ounces each)
2 tablespoons Italian breadcrumbs
2 teaspoons extra-virgin olive oil
¾ cup prepared salsa
½ diced plum tomato
½ cup diced zucchini
2 tablespoons seedless Kalamata olives
2 teaspoons capers

Pound chicken breast between sheets of wax paper to a uniform ½-inch thickness. Sprinkle with breadcrumbs.

Heat oil in a large skillet and sauté chicken until golden, about 2 minutes on each side. Add a splash of water, cover, and cook until done through, about 6 minutes.

Stir salsa, tomato, zucchini, olives, and capers together.

To serve, arrange chicken on a plate and top with salsa.

Nutritional readout: CALORIES 245, FAT 5.1 g., PROTEIN 40.1 g., CARBS 5.3 g., FIBER .6 g.

Easy-roast Chicken Thighs and Asparagus

Simple and satisfying, this one-dish dinner goes together in a hurry. And check out the carb count, fewer than 8.

Makes 4 servings

2 garlic cloves
Salt
Freshly grated black pepper
3 tablespoons extra-virgin olive oil, divided
2 tablespoons fresh lemon juice, divided
8 chicken thighs with skin (about 1¾ pounds)
2 tablespoons unsalted butter, divided
½ cup chicken broth
12 spears asparagus
1 teaspoon fresh or dried oregano
Parsley for garnish
Lemon wedges for garnish

Preheat oven to 450°F. Mince garlic with a pinch of salt. Then whisk together with ½ teaspoon salt, ¼ teaspoon pepper, 2 tablespoons oil, and 1 tablespoon lemon juice. Pat chicken dry and coat with lemon-garlic mixture.

Heat 1 tablespoon butter and remaining oil in a 12-inch heavy skillet over medium-high heat and brown chicken in two batches, skin side down, until golden and crisp; then remove to a baking dish, skin side up. Arrange asparagus alongside chicken. Pour off fat from skillet. Add broth and remaining tablespoon lemon juice and boil until reduced by half, about 2 minutes. Whisk in remaining tablespoon butter and oregano, and then pour over chicken and asparagus.

Roast chicken in oven until cooked through, about 20 minutes. Add a grating of freshly milled black pepper and serve, garnished with parsley and lemon wedges.

Nutritional Readout: CALORIES 467, FAT 33.3 g., PROTEIN 35.6 g., CARBS 7.8 g., FIBER 1.3 g.

Chicken Thighs in a Mushroom Sauce

Meatier thighs have a great flavor, and if you buy them boneless and skinless, they are oh so easy to deal with. On the table in under 15.

Makes 4 servings

2 cups chicken broth
¼ cup tomato paste
1 teaspoon dried rubbed sage
Kosher salt to taste
Freshly milled black pepper to taste
4 skinless, boneless chicken thighs
4 teaspoons Italian-seasoned breadcrumbs
1 tablespoon extra-virgin olive oil
½ pound sliced baby bella mushrooms
4 green onions, thinly sliced on the diagonal

Combine broth with tomato paste, sage, salt, and pepper. Set aside.

Sprinkle chicken with additional salt and pepper and then breadcrumbs. Heat oil in a large skillet and cook chicken 2–3 minutes per side. Add mushroom and brown them for 2 minutes; then add broth mixture. Cover and cook until chicken is done, about 10 minutes. Sprinkle with green onions and serve.

Nutritional readout: CALORIES 260, FAT 4.9 g., PROTEIN 44.1 g., CARBS 9.2 g., FIBER 2.2 g.

Feta-stuffed Chicken

Feta is a full-flavored cheese that can be used in small amounts. Here it is mixed with a little cream cheese (lowering the carbohydrate content even more) and used as a stuffing for chicken.

Makes 4 servings

¼ cup crumbled basil-and-tomato feta cheese (1 ounce)*
2 tablespoons (1 ounce) cream cheese
4 skinless, boneless chicken breast halves (about 1¼ pounds total)
Dash sea salt
¼ to ½ teaspoon black pepper
1 teaspoon extra-virgin olive oil
¼ cup chicken broth
1 10-ounce package prewashed fresh spinach, trimmed
2 tablespoons walnut or pecan pieces, toasted
1 tablespoon lemon juice
Lemon slices, halved (optional)

In a small bowl, combine feta cheese and cream cheese; set aside.

Using a sharp knife, cut a horizontal slit through the thickest portion of each chicken breast half to form a pocket. Stuff pockets with the cheese mixture. If necessary, secure openings with wooden toothpicks. Sprinkle chicken with pepper and salt.

In a large nonstick skillet, cook chicken in hot oil over medium-high heat about 12 minutes or until tender and no longer pink, turning once (reduce heat to medium if chicken browns too quickly). Remove chicken from skillet. Cover and keep warm.

Carefully add chicken broth to skillet. Bring to boiling and add half of the spinach. Cover and cook about 3 minutes or just until spinach is wilted. Remove spinach from skillet, reserving liquid in pan. Repeat with remaining spinach. Return all spinach to skillet. Stir in the nuts and lemon juice.

To serve, divide spinach mixture among 4 dinner plates. Top with chicken breasts. If desired, garnish with lemon slices.

*Note: If basil-and-tomato feta cheese is not available, stir 1 teaspoon finely snipped fresh basil and 1 teaspoon snipped oil-pack dried tomatoes, drained, into ¼ cup plain feta cheese.

Nutrition Readout: CALORIES 231, FAT 8 g., PROTEIN 38 g., CARBS 2 g., FIBER 6 g.

Thanksgiving Turkey with Low-carb Stuffing

Yes, Virginia, it is possible to create a low-carb turkey stuffing that will taste just as good as Grandmother's old-fashioned dish made with biscuits, cornbread, and/or bread. The trick is to find a suitable substitute for all of that forbidden starch.

Shirataki noodles are the answer. (You can order shiritaki noodles from www.MiracleNoodle.com or pick them up at your local Chinese grocery.) They are amazing. Calorie- and carb-free, they pick up the flavors around them, so when stuffed into the bird with all of the other great veggies, it is just stupendous. Happy Turkey Day.

This recipe with only a turkey breast works great for small families. You could also stuff a whole turkey, in which case, DOUBLE the stuffing ingredients. All good.

Make sure you begin this the day before.

Makes 6–8 servings

1 5-pound boned and butterflied organic turkey breast with skin (get the butcher to do this)
Brine
½ bottle white wine
Water to cover
1 cup kosher salt
2 bay leaves
3–4 peppercorns
Stuffing
Extra-virgin olive oil
Butter to film the pan and to drizzle over the turkey
1 large yellow onion, minced
3 celery ribs with leaves, minced
Poultry seasoning
1 bay leaf
1 pound sweet Italian sausage, removed from casing and crumbled
5 brown mushrooms, chopped

½ cup walnut pieces
¼ cup dried cranberries
1 pound shirataki noodles, rinsed and chopped
2 large eggs, beaten
Sea salt to taste
Freshly cracked black pepper to taste
Olive oil

Begin brining the turkey the day before. Place it in a large pan; add white wine and enough water to cover and then salt, bay leaves, and peppercorns. Cover and refrigerate overnight.

When you are ready to cook, remove the turkey to the counter and pat dry with paper towels.

Meanwhile, heat a 12-inch heavy skillet with olive oil and butter. Began sweating the onion. Add celery, a bay leaf, sprinkling of poultry seasoning and let it go a few minutes. While that is cooking over medium-low heat, toss the crumbled sausage into the skillet. Turn the fire up to brown the meat. Add the mushrooms, walnuts, and cranberries.

Rinse the shiritaki noodles, cut them with scissors, and toss into the mix, letting the noodles cook a bit. Adjust the seasonings with sea salt and cracked black pepper. Take it off the heat to cool.

Finally mix the eggs with the cooled stuffing ingredients.

Lay out the turkey breast and whack it with a pounder under wax paper until it is a fairly uniform ½-inch thick. Spread the stuffing on top, leaving a narrow band around the edges Roll it up, tie it with kitchen string in three or four places, and put it into an oiled Le Creuset baking dish.

Put the stuffed turkey in a 375°F oven, dab it with melted butter, and let it roast until the thermometer registers 155°. The whole kitchen will smell great. Take it out, rest it a bit, cut and discard the strings, then take it to the table with accoutrements—green beans, cranberry relish, and fresh pumpkin and ginger pickle. Yum.

Nutritional readout: CALORIES 460, FAT 34 g., PROTEIN 35.6 g., CARBS 7.2 g., FIBER 1.2 g.

Basil-parsley Chicken Salad

Feel free to toss in other leafy greens of your choice, celery leaves, baby spinach, and mixed greens. This is a yummy lunch served over a bed of spring greens or wrapped in a butter-lettuce leaf.

Makes 4 servings

1½ cup cooked chicken, chopped
¼ cup basil, cut chiffonade
½ cup minced celery
¼ cup minced green onion
¼ cup chopped Italian parsley
2 tablespoons chopped sweet red peppers
½ cup mayonnaise
2 tablespoons Greek yogurt
Kosher salt to taste
Freshly milled black pepper to taste

Mix ingredients in a medium bowl, cover, and refrigerate. Serve on a bed of spring greens or in a lettuce wrap.

Nutritional readout: CALORIES 165, FAT 7.2 g., PROTEIN 20 g., CARBS 3.8 g., FIBER .7 g.

Hotcha Flank Steak

Cook the whole thing in less than 10 minutes and feed 8 people once, or 1 person 8 times.

Makes 8 servings

2 pounds flank steak
Kosher salt to taste
Cracked black pepper to taste
¼ cup fresh lime juice
Grated zest from 1 lime
2 tablespoons extra-virgin olive oil
6 cloves garlic, smashed
1 teaspoon (or to taste) crushed red pepper
½ teaspoon salt
Lime wedges for garnish

Score flank steak and put it in a ziplock bag. Add remaining ingredients, zip it up, and marinate 30 minutes on the counter or up to 8 hours in the refrigerator.

When ready to cook, heat the grill and cook 4–5 minutes on each side. Rest on a cutting board and then cut into thin slices. Serve, garnished with additional lime wedges.

Nutritional readout. CALORIES 189, FAT 8.9 g., PROTEIN 24.8 g., CARBS 1.3 g., FIBER 0.1 g.

Hoisin Beef Stir-fry with Asparagus and Sweet Bell Peppers

Just like going out to eat where you ask them to leave the rice to the side, here, you just serve this in a bowl and enjoy it without any additional carbs.

Makes 6 servings ready to serve in less than 10 minutes

2 tablespoons soy sauce, divided
1 tablespoon cornstarch, divided
1 pound boneless beef steak, cut into ½-inch strips
½ cup chicken broth
2 tablespoons hoisin sauce
1 tablespoon rice vinegar
1 teaspoon dark sesame oil
¼ teaspoon crushed red pepper
¼ cup sesame oil, divided
1 red or orange bell pepper, sliced thin
1 pound asparagus, cut into 2-inch pieces
1 green onion, thinly sliced
1 tablespoon sesame seeds, white or black

Combine 1 tablespoon soy sauce and ½ tablespoon cornstarch in a bowl. Whisk until smooth. Add beef, rubbing mixture into all surfaces.
Combine remaining soy sauce and cornstarch, broth, hoisin, rice vinegar, dark oil, and crushed red pepper.
Heat 2 teaspoons sesame oil in a large skillet and sauté beef, stirring, about 5 minutes or until lightly browned. Remove to a warm bowl. Add remaining oil to skillet and stir-fry the bell pepper, asparagus, and green onion until crisp tender. Add beef and broth mixture and cook until hot through, about 30 seconds. Serve at once, sprinkled with sesame seeds.
Nutritional readout: CALORIES 243, FAT 14.6 g., PROTEIN 17.3 g., CARBS 10.6 g., FIBER 2 g.

Stilton Beef with Sherry-mushroom Sauce

Have a reason to celebrate? Now you do. Add a side of roasted asparagus, and it's a party.

Makes 4 4-ounce servings

4 4-ounce beef tenderloins (filet mignon)
Kosher salt to taste
Cracked black pepper to taste
2 tablespoons extra-virgin olive oil
½ pound sliced, mixed forest mushrooms
1 cup dry sherry
¼ cup Worcestershire sauce
1 packet sugar substitute
1 teaspoon fresh oregano
1 ounce (¼ cup) crumbled Stilton (or other blue) cheese for
    garnish
¼ cup chopped fresh parsley for garnish

Season beef with salt and pepper. Heat a large skillet over medium-high heat and sear steaks about 3 minutes per side for medium. Add mushrooms once you turn the meat.

Meanwhile, combine sherry, Worcestershire sauce, sugar substitute, and oregano.

Remove steaks to a warm plate and cover. Add sherry mixture to the pan and reduce by half. Serve steaks with mushrooms and sauce, sprinkled with Stilton and parsley.

Nutritional readout: CALORIES 295, FAT 11.3 g., PROTEIN 26 g., CARBS 7.8 g., FIBER .8 g.

Roast Pork Loin with Dry-cured Olives

Another dish that repays you with great leftovers for lunch, this luxurious-looking dish is easy to prepare and rewarding to serve.
Makes 10 servings

1 boneless pork loin (4 to 6 pounds)
½ cup seedless dry-cured black olives
2 cloves garlic, slivered
1 teaspoon rosemary needles
Freshly milled black pepper to taste
1 tablespoon extra-virgin olive oil
1 cup veal or beef stock
1 cup dry white wine
1 cup pork skins, crushed
1 tablespoon Madeira
Parsley for garnish

Heat oven to 400°F.

Cut deeply into the pork loin, lengthwise, to open up a flap. Then add olives, garlic, rosemary, and pepper. Roll and tie the roast at 1-inch intervals using cotton string. Heat oil in a large roasting pan in the oven, and then add the meat and brown for 15 minutes.

Meanwhile, heat stock and wine, then pour over the meat, reduce heat to 325°F, and continue roasting until meat reaches an internal temperature of 140°F. Remove roast to a serving platter to rest. Add pork skins to pan juices and stir and boil to make a sauce. Add Madeira to sauce; then taste and adjust seasonings. Garnish with parsley. Slice thin and pass the gravy.

Nutritional readout: CALORIES 422, FAT 20.5 g., PROTEIN 48.8 g., CARBS 5.3 g., FIBER .1 g.

Five-spice Lamb Chops with Raspberry Salsa

Quick as a wink and brightly flavored.

Makes 4 servings

8 trimmed lamb chops
2 teaspoons five-spice powder
Salt to taste
Freshly milled black pepper to taste
2 cups fresh raspberries
1 teaspoon freshly grated ginger root
1 packet sugar substitute
2 teaspoons rice wine vinegar
2 tablespoons extra-virgin olive oil

Season pork with five-spice, salt, and pepper.

Make salsa by combining raspberries, ginger, sugar substitute, and rice wine vinegar in a bowl.

Heat oil in a large skillet and cook meat, about 2 minutes to the side or until golden. Mound salsa over chops to serve.

Nutritional readout: CALORIES 220, FAT 9.2 g., PROTEIN 24 g., CARBS 10 g., FIBER 1.7 g.

Parvathy Ramachandran's Eggplant-chickpea Gravy

Keep a pot of this luscious South Indian-style sauce in the refrigerator and spoon it over cooked chicken or fish for a fantastic, flavorful one-dish dinner.

Makes 10 servings

> 4 tablespoons olive or sesame oil (choose sesame for the South Indian flavor)
> 1 tablespoon cumin seeds
> 1 teaspoon turmeric powder
> 1 large garlic clove, peeled and smashed
> 1 piece fresh ginger, about 1x2 inches, peeled and minced
> ½ small green or red hot pepper (optional) seeded, minced
> 1 small red onion, peeled and finely chopped
> 2 tablespoons garam masala OR madras curry powder, dissolved in 2 tablespoons water
> 1 medium eggplant, chopped and salted with 1 teaspoon kosher salt
> 1 14-ounce can chopped tomatoes and juice
> 1 16-ounce can chickpeas, drained
> ½ cup fresh cilantro, chopped

Heat the oil in a large skillet. Add cumin seeds and turmeric and allow to sputter, about 30 seconds. Add the garlic, ginger, hot pepper (if using), and onion and cook over medium heat, stirring, until the onion is clear, about 3 to 5 minutes. Add garam masala or curry powder mixed in water. Stir vigorously, then add eggplant, and cook until it begins to brown and soften, about 5 minutes. Add tomatoes and chickpeas and cook 10 minutes or so, tasting and adjusting salt as needed. Toss in cilantro at the end. Serve over meat, fish, or ¼ cup basmati rice, white or brown.

Nutritional readout: CALORIES 282, FAT 16.6 g., PROTEIN 25.1 g., CARBS 8.2 g., FIBER 3.2 g.

St. Croix Curry

The Indian Diaspora took curry to the Caribbean where it found a welcome home. You can almost hear the calypso beat when you cook this. Although goat is the meat of choice, you can substitute fish, veal, beef, lamb, or even chicken. The flavor is intense and satisfying. The work is minimal. You will love it. Skip the traditional rice until you have come within 5 pounds of your goal weight.

Makes 8 servings

2 pounds boneless stew meat (veal, beef, lamb, chicken, or goat)
Kosher salt
Freshly milled black pepper
2 tablespoons coconut oil (or olive oil)
1 large red onion, finely chopped
2 garlic cloves, crushed
1 tablespoon (or more to taste) hot curry powder
½ teaspoon ground cumin
½ teaspoon crushed red pepper (or to taste)
2 cups chicken broth
Juice and zest from 4 limes
½ cup minced green onions for garnish

Season meat generously with salt and pepper. Heat oil in a large, deep stew pot, and then brown the meat, a few pieces at a time. Add onion and garlic and heat about a minute; then stir in curry powder, cumin, and red pepper. Heat another minute; then add broth and simmer until meat is tender, about 1 hour. Stir in lime juice and zest and serve, topped with green onions.

For those who have come within 5 pounds of goal weight, add ½ cup cooked brown rice to the bottom of your soup bowl and spoon curry on top.

Nutritional readout: CALORIES 252, FAT 15 g., PROTEIN 24 g., CARBS 5.2 g., FIBER .9 g.

Bacon, Sausage, and Cabbage Soup

The secret to the success of this soup is the method. Take your time, "sweat" the vegetables in order just until they have begun to glisten and turn brown before adding one drop of liquid, and the flavor will simply leap out at you.

Makes 8 1-cup servings

4 strips thick bacon, chopped
1 6-inch link low-fat kielbasa, cut into coins
3 celery sticks
2 medium onions
½ red or yellow bell pepper
6 garlic cloves
1-inch piece of fresh ginger
1 tablespoon curry powder (or more to suit)
Grated zest of 1 orange
1 small head Savoy or other cabbage
Kosher salt to taste
Freshly ground black pepper to taste
1 quart chicken broth
1 14½-ounce can diced tomatoes and juice
Sour cream for garnish
Minced cilantro and/or fresh jalapeno for garnish

In a large soup pot over medium heat, begin to cook bacon and kielbasa.

Meanwhile, place slicing disk on the food processor. Slice thinly each of the vegetables IN ORDER, and as you complete each one, add it to the pot: celery, onions, bell pepper, garlic, ginger. Add the curry and orange zest and then thinly slice the cabbage and add it to the pot. Take your time. Let the vegetables cook down. Stir and do not rush.

Add salt and pepper and then the broth and tomatoes. By the time you add the broth and tomatoes, the vegetables should have cooked down by half their volume. Cover the pot and cook about 15 minutes.

Serve in bowls, garnished with sour cream and cilantro.

Nutritional readout: CALORIES 87, FAT 4.7 g., PROTEIN 3.1 g., CARBS 9.4 g., FIBER 2.4 g.

Kale with Garlic and Bacon

Quick to fix and deeply satisfying.

Makes 4 servings

1½ pounds kale (about 2 bunches), tough stems and center
    ribs cut off and discarded
10 bacon slices (½ pound), cut into ½-inch pieces
4 garlic cloves, finely chopped
½ teaspoon (or to taste) red chili flakes
1 cup chicken broth
Salt to taste
Freshly milled black pepper to taste

Stack a few kale leaves and roll lengthwise into a cigar shape. Cut crosswise into ¼-inch-wide strips with a sharp knife. Repeat with remaining leaves.

Cook bacon in a wide 6- to 8-quart, heavy pot over moderate heat, stirring occasionally, until crisp; then transfer with a slotted spoon to paper towels to drain. Cook garlic and red chili in remaining fat over moderately low heat, stirring, until pale golden, about 30 seconds. Add kale (pot will be full) and cook, turning with tongs, until wilted and bright green, about 1 minute. Add broth and simmer, partially covered, until just tender, 6 to 10 minutes. Toss with bacon and salt and pepper to taste.

Nutritional Readout: CALORIES 375, FAT 26 g., PROTEIN 22.31 g., CARBS 18.1 g., FIBER 1.36 g.

Dijon Salmon with Bacon and Pecans

Makes 8 servings

1 filet wild salmon (approximately 1½ pounds)
3 tablespoons melted, unsalted butter
3 tablespoons agave syrup
3 tablespoons Dijon mustard
¾ cup chopped pecans
Salt and pepper to taste
6 slices Boss Hog's No-Nitrite Hickory-Smoked Country Bacon,
    cooked and chopped

Preheat oven to 400°F. Mix melted butter, agave syrup, and Dijon mustard in a small bowl. Season salmon filet with salt and pepper. Spread mixture evenly on the salmon and then top with the chopped pecans.

Place in oven and bake for 10 minutes per 1-inch thickness of salmon until done and no longer translucent and fish flakes easily. Do not overcook. Sprinkle chopped, cooked bacon on fish; serve and enjoy!

Approximate Nutritional Readout: CALORIES 289, FAT 20 g., PROTEIN 20 g., CARBS 8 g., FIBER 1 g.

This original recipe comes from Bacontoday.com

Bacon-wrapped Brussels Sprouts

Makes 16 servings

1 pound Boss Hog's No-Nitrite Pepper County Bacon
1 pound Brussels sprouts
2 tablespoons extra-virgin olive oil
2 tablespoons Dijon mustard
Toothpicks that have been soaked in water
    (to avoid burning)

Preheat oven to 400°F. Wash Brussels sprouts and trim the brown stems. Pat dry and add to a large mixing bowl. Cut large sprouts in half lengthwise.

Mix olive oil and Dijon in a small bowl. Pour the marinade over the sprouts and toss to combine.

Cut bacon so it will just fit around the sprout. Wrap bacon around each Brussels sprout, securing with a toothpick.

Line a rimmed baking sheet with foil. Assemble sprouts green-side down. Cook for approximately 25–30 minutes, turning the sprouts over halfway through. Sprouts are done when the bacon is crispy and cooked. If you have more sprouts than bacon, add them to the pan with the bacon grease and roast in the fat for 25–30 minutes, turning occasionally.

Let cool for 5 minutes before eating, as the sprouts will be very hot.

Approximate Nutritional Readout: CALORIES 154, FAT 13 g., PROTEIN 4 g., CARBS 2 g., FIBER .1 g.

This original recipe comes from Bacontoday.com

Curried Roasted Cauliflower with Bacon

Makes 6 servings

1 head of cauliflower
2-3 tablespoons olive oil
1 teaspoon curry powder
Salt and pepper to taste
6 slices Boss Hog No-Nitrite Hickory-Smoked Bacon,
    cooked and chopped

Chop cauliflower into florets. Mix olive oil, curry powder, and salt and pepper. Toss the florets in the olive oil mixture until coated.

Preheat oven to 425°F. Roast cauliflower for 20-25 minutes or until tender, turning occasionally to avoid burning.

Top with crumbled, cooked bacon bits and serve.

Approximate Nutritional Readout: CALORIES 144, FAT 12 g., PROTEIN 7 g., CARBS 5 g., FIBER 2.5 g.

This original recipe comes from Bacontoday.com

Texas Caviar

Party fave for footballers, this healthy topping can lift a chicken breast, slice of pork roast, or fish fillet to new heights.

Makes 20 ¼-cup servings

3 tablespoons chopped fresh cilantro
3 tablespoons red wine vinegar
2 tablespoons extra-virgin olive oil
Hot sauce to taste, shake it on good
1 garlic clove, smashed
2 15.8-ounce cans black-eyed peas, rinsed and drained
1½ cups diced red onion
1 cup diced seeded tomato
1 cup diced red, green, and/or yellow bell pepper

Toss all ingredients together in a large bowl. Cover and refrigerate.

Nutritional readout: CALORIES 43, FAT 1.6 g., PROTEIN 1.7 g., CARBS 5.8 g., FIBER 1.4 g.

Summer Fruit Salsa

Spoon over no-sugar-added ice cream or custard for a divine dessert.
Makes 12 ¼-cup servings

1½ cups chopped cantaloupe
1 cup chopped pineapple
½ cup craisins (dried cranberries)
½ cup chopped fresh mint
2 tablespoons fresh lemon juice
Grated zest from 1 lemon
1 teaspoon grated fresh ginger root
1 small jalapeno, seeded and minced

Combine ingredients in a bowl, cover, and refrigerate.

Nutritional Readout: CALORIES 29, FAT 0.1 g., PROTEIN .3 g.,
CARBS 7.7 g., FIBER .6 g.

Bloody Mary Shrimp Dipper

OK. Go ahead and drink it out of the cup. It is that good and only 4.6 grams of carbs per ¼ cup serving. But, really, bathe cold boiled shrimp, oysters on the half shell, or clams with this zesty flavor.

Makes 8 ¼-cup servings

1 cup thick Bloody Mary Cocktail mix
½ cup finely chopped sweet onion
½ cup minced cilantro
½ cup minced celery
½ cup chopped berry tomato
½ cup chopped celery leaves
Big shot of Worcestershire sauce
Big shot of Tabasco sauce

Combine all ingredients in a bowl, cover, and refrigerate.

Nutritional readout: CALORIES 20, FAT .1 g., PROTEIN .5 g., CARBS 4.6 g., FIBER .8 g.

APPENDIX

The proposed 2010 Dietary Guidelines continue the misguided shibboleths against saturated fats and animal foods rich in nutrient dense fatty acids, including egg yolks, butter, cream, whole milk, cheese and fatty meats including bacon as well as animal fats for cooking. In my 20 year practice of medicine in New York City, I have treated many patients whose health had been severely compromised by excluding these necessary nutrients in their daily diet. It is my experience, backed up by scientific studies, that low fat diets have caused many of today's lifestyle ailments including obesity, diabetes, heart disease and stroke.

Basic biochemistry shows that the human body has a high requirement for saturated fats in the cell membranes, brain and other organs. If we do not eat saturated fats, the body makes fat from refined carbohydrates, leading to rapid weight gain and chronic illness.

The proposed guidelines will exacerbate existing nutrient deficiencies that I see in my practice every day. Common deficiencies in vitamins A, D, K2 and E which are found in animal fats, vitamins B12 and B6, found in animal foods, as well as minerals including iron, calcium and zinc which require vitamins A and D for assimilation. It is my experience that these deficiencies can be easily corrected by a proper diet of whole foods, organic if possible, with naturally occurring animal fats.

I have seen, in my practice, children as young as 8 years old, suffering from type 2 diabetes, an ailment that used to be seen only in later middle age. Why are these children getting diabetes? Low fat milk, soy milk, apple juice, too many processed carbohydrates, and insufficient natural animal fats. Fortunately, type 2 diabetes can be stopped in its tracks by a radical shift in the diet. Give those children whole milk, plenty of protein and natural animal fats, get the sugars out of their diets, and their diabetes will correct itself, their weight will normalize and they will be healthy.

Our misguided dietary public policy has created a society of very sick people. For the first time in history we see a generation who may not live as long as its parents.

Particularly in the lower classes without access to healthy, whole foods, we are creating a society of people who will not be well, who will require huge public assistance and health care, and all of it could be alleviated by a proper diet.

From the viewpoint of a practicing physician, I can tell you that our industrial food complex, in concert with big pharma have colluded to create a society where people eat nutrient-empty processed foods, and are than given an ever larger regimen of pharmaceuticals to try and turn back the inevitable ill health and death that awaits them.

Besides the fact that our enormously powerful industrial food/ farming lobby has exercised great control over public policy for at least twenty years, since I have been observing it, the results, in the time that I have been practicing medicine, have been dreadful.

When I was a boy, growing up in an Italian American family, my grandfather had a big vegetable garden out back that fed our family. He lived to be ninety-five years old and was strong and active until the day he died. I try to feed my family, whole, organic foods to this day. My six year old son, rides with me in bicycle races for as much as 45 miles at a time. This child is healthy, vigorous, and cheerful. He gets whole milk, plenty of butter and red meat, and a good assortment of whole organic fruits and vegetables.

Is it impossible that Americans could eat as well as their grandparents? Not at all. With the growing movement towards healthier whole foods being presented not only at home, but in public schools, institutions, and food service operations, Americans are beginning to get it.

At The Fight Fat with Fat Diet we particularly recognize the need for saturated fats, for health, long life, and weight loss. Saturated fats fight inflammation, support the immune system, support hormone production and protect against cancer and heart disease.

Last but not least what I see in my practice that is most heartbreaking is the rising tide of infertility. Now that we have an entire generation of young women who have practically grown up eating a low fat diet, we see a pandemic of infertility. The simple truth is that vitamins carried in saturated animal fats are critical to reproduction. The 2010 Guidelines proposed by the USDA will increase infertility in this country. This is tragic and entirely avoidable.

The knee-jerk recommendation to eat more whole grains, does not take into account the fact that whole grains are extremely difficult to digest and an overconsumption of rough whole grains can contribute to digestive disorders such as celiac disease and irritable bowel syndrome.

The Fight Fat with Fat Diet recommends that people eat a diet of whole, unprocessed foods, organic if possible, that provide an abundance of nutrients chosen from the following groups:

1. Animal foods: meat and organ meats, poultry and eggs from pastured animals, wild caught fish and shell fish,

whole raw cheeses, milk and other dairy products from pastured animals.

2. Fats and oils: unrefined saturated and monounsaturated fats including butter, lard, olive oil, cod liver oil and coconut and palm oil.

3. Fruits and Vegetables. Fresh, organic if possible, preferably locally grown, either raw or cooked into soups and stews

4. Nuts, legumes, and grains. Eat a handful of nuts daily for vitamin E and trace minerals. Once goal weight is reached eat beans and lentils, brown rice, and whole grain cooked cereals for breakfast.

We do not recommend processed foods with long lists of ingredient including chemicals you cannot pronounce. No refined sweeteners including candy, soda, cookies, crackers, cakes, chips or other snacks. Avoid white flour products such as pasta and white bread. Avoid processed foods including modern soy foods, polyunsaturated and partially hydrogenated vegetable oils and fried foods.

As we say at the Fight Fat with Fat Diet, take a giant leap backwards. Eat the way your grandparents ate. You take care of your body and your body will take care of you.

INDEX

RECIPE INDEX

ABOUT THE AUTHOR

DR. JOHN P. SALERNO

Board Certified, American Board of Family Practice

Lauded as an international pioneer in the field of anti-aging, Dr. John P. Salerno is a leader in the practice of complementary medicine. Based in Manhattan, Dr. Salerno has been cited as an expert by national media outlets, retained as a consultant by world-renowned medical luminaries for the launching of treatment facilities across three continents, and referenced by Suzanne Somers in her #1 New York Times bestseller, *Ageless*, and in her 2009 follow-ups, *Breakthrough: Eight Steps to Wellness* and *Knockout*. Somers told an audience in 2006, "I will personally send patients to Dr. Salerno."

Dr. Salerno is the founder of the Salerno Center for Complementary Medicine, established in New York City in 2005. He is also the co-founder of anti-aging clinics in Tokyo and the chief medical officer behind the RenuLife anti-aging and dermatological clinic in Sao Paolo, Brazil.

Best known for his weight-loss treatments, bio-identical hormone replacement, vitamin IV suites, and chelation therapy, a process that removes heavy metals from the body, Dr. Salerno lists dozens of celebrities among his patients. He combines the teachings of traditional medicine with the wisdom of alternative healing to cleanse the system of toxins and blockages that can cause heart disease, cancer, brain dysfunction, diabetes, and others. He boosts the body's immune system with products chosen from a line of natural vita-nutrients that he created in conjunction with Dr. Hiroyuki Abe, president of the International Society of Integrative Medicine and owner of the Kudan Clinic in Japan.

Dr. Salerno is a licensed physician in the State of New York and in Florida. Dr. Salerno served three years as clinical preceptor at the Yale University School of Medicine. He is also a diplomate of the National Board of Osteopathic Medical Examiners, a board certified member of the American Osteopathic Board of Family Practice, and member in good standing of the American Osteopathic Association, the American College for Advancement in Medicine, the American Medical Association, and the American Academy of Anti-Aging Medicine.

Dr. Salerno graduated magna cum laude from Adelphi University, where he earned a Bachelor of Science in biology, and received his Doctor of Osteopathic Medicine degree from New York College of Osteopathic Medicine of New York Institute of Technology. He completed his internship and family-practice residency at New York's Long Beach Medical Center, during which time he conducted lab research at Columbia University Medical Center.

ABOUT THE SALERNO CENTER

At the Salerno Center for Complementary Medicine, the physician-patient relationship is an important part of our practice. As a dedicated healthcare provider, we know each person has an important story, set of treatment guidelines, and health principles. Because of the nature of our body's related systems, illness is a dysfunction of the whole person, which is why Dr. Salerno's primary goal is to balance the physical, mental, and lifestyle factors that define healthy living.

By using natural medicine as a foundation and modern diagnostic testing techniques to detect any abnormalities, Dr. Salerno is able to accurately pinpoint and treat the root cause(s) of the individual's health problem. In order to prevent future outbreaks from occurring, Dr. Salerno emphasizes health education and self-empowerment, which allow his patients to make healthy choices on a daily basis.

Bio-identical Hormone Replacement Therapy (BHRT)

Among the many services the Salerno Center provides is bio-identical hormone replacement therapy. BHRT treats the symptoms of menopause, perimenopause, and postmenopause. Those symptoms can include hot flashes, bloating, weight gain, mood swings, and brain fog.

BHRT is not to be confused with synthetic hormone treatment, like the horse urine tabs that jolted a woman's body with enormous doses of estrogen and subjected her body to an increased risk for cancer of the breast and female organs. The synthetics in those have been named in warnings by the FDA as dangerous to women's health and adding significant risk for female organ cancers.

On the contrary, BHRT ingredients are molecularly identical to endogenous hormones in the woman's body and are compounded for us in our own pharmacy.

In BHRT, first, we evaluate each woman's condition through an intake exam and complete blood work. Once we determine that a woman's natural hormones are in decline, either from menopause, or even hysterectomy, we begin a regimen of BHRT. We determine the exact mix for each woman and compound a blend of estrone, estradiol, and progesterone, as well as testosterone. (Yes, women need a bit of testosterone, too!) In a case-by-case determination, we may add pregnenolone, dehydroepiandrosterone (DHEA), and estriol, which, to date, are not approved for use in Canada or the United States but are widely used in Europe, Asia, and South America by us and many other medical practitioners. In addition to stabilizing a woman's moods and reducing or eliminating night sweats and hot flashes, BHRT reduces the risk of osteoporosis and can help postmenopausal women who are having trouble losing weight.

After putting a woman on a regimen of BHRT, we do periodic blood work and may adjust the dosage, based on the results.

Results of BHRT

My BHRT protocols are used not only in my New York practice but also in practices I supervise in Japan and Brazil. BHRT is key to anti-aging issues and is, in my experience, intertwined with weight issues in postmenopausal women.

Suzanne Somers, author of *Ageless, Breakthrough: Eight Steps to Wellness*, and *Knockout*, highly recommends BHRT. Oprah also joins me in understanding the miraculous results from designing a BHRT plan for each woman. Both Suzanne Somers and Oprah are enthusiastic users of BHRT.

We find BHRT to be an enormous asset to women clients, forty-five to eighty, on the Fight Fat with Fat Diet, and we use it judiciously at the Salerno Centers worldwide. The Fight Fat with Fat Diet is ideal for women because it focuses on high-quality protein and natural fats with plenty of fresh vegetables and fruits. We recommend supplements as well, but sometimes hormone imbalances must be addressed, and that is when we turn to BHRT.

Supplements

The Salerno Center offers various beneficial supplements as an insurance policy for good health. The section, "The Importance of Supplements" itemizes those we can provide to our clients.

Our office patients may elect to receive supplements by weekly IV infusions. We also prescribe pure, organic supplements and compounds made especially for our patients and for our website readers (www.thesilverclouddiet.com).

To learn more about The Salerno Center, call 1-212-582-1700. Of course, you are always welcome to become a patient of The Salerno Center, located at 161 Madison Avenue, New York, New York. We have years of experience and great success in treating weight loss and other conditions, including candida.